Seeing Without Glasses

A Step-by-Step Approach to Improving Eyesight Naturally

THIRD EDITION

Roberto Kaplan, O.D., M.Ed.

BEYOND
WORDS
Publishing
I N C

Beyond Words Publishing, Inc.
20827 N.W. Cornell Road, Suite 500
Hillsboro, Oregon 97124-9808
503-531-8700

First published in 1987 as *Seeing Beyond 20/20*
Second edition 1994 as *Seeing Without Glasses: Improving Your Vision Naturally*
Third edition 2003

The information contained in this book is intended to be educational and not for diagnosis, prescription, or treatment of eye conditions or disease or any health disorder whatsoever. This information should not replace competent optometric or medical care. The content of the book is intended to be used as an adjunct to a rational and responsible vision-care program prescribed by an eye doctor. The author and publisher are in no way liable for any use or mis-use of the material. The case studies in this book are real; however, the names have been changed.

Editor: Julie Livingston
Proofreader: Marvin Moore
Illustrator: Suellen Larkin
Design: Principia Graphica and Connie Lightner
Composition: William H. Brunson Typography Services

Printed in the United States of America
Distributed to the book trade by Publishers Group West

Library of Congress Cataloging-in-Publication Data
Kaplan, Robert-Michael.
    Seeing without glasses : a step-by-step approach to improving eyesight naturally / Roberto Kaplan.— 3rd ed.
      p. cm.
    Previously published in 1994 with subtitle : improving your vision naturally.
    Includes bibliographical references.
    ISBN 1-58270-089-3
    1. Vision disorders—Alternative treatment.   2. Vision disorders—Prevention.   3. Vision disorders—Nutritional aspects.   4. Orthoptics.
5. Naturopathy.   6. Visual training.   I. Title.
    RE48 .K33   2003
    617.7—dc21

                  2002153413

The corporate mission of Beyond Words Publishing, Inc.:
  Inspire to Integrity

Seeing Without Glasses

To all of you who have reminded me
to look from the heart, thank you

Contents

Part 4: Clearer Vision

Preface

Seeing Without Glasses has been researched and tested for over fifteen years. This third edition includes two new chapters: "Using Pinholes to Improve Your Vision" and "Help for Eye-Disease Conditions." What began in 1982 as a clinical investigation into whether nearsightedness can actually be corrected has resulted in a profound vision-fitness training program for eye disease and nearsighted, farsighted, and astigmatic conditions for adults and children.

At first I believed that improving eyesight was just a matter of doing some exercises like calisthenics. During the past thirty-two years my patients have taught me that enhancing vision requires a holistic approach. Many aspects of an individual's lifestyle need to be examined.

For this reason, I wrote a new book called *Conscious Seeing* (Beyond Words Publishing, 2002). Where *Seeing Without Glasses* gives you the practical steps for improving your physical eyesight, *Conscious Seeing* helps you delve into the exciting realm of inner vision.

Seeing more deeply into life begins behind the eye, in the brain and mind. Read together, these two books demonstrate that the most important step in improving your eyesight is to begin seeing differently.

Take off your glasses and spend time in nature in your naked vision. Obtain weaker glasses and start a daily program of practices that will help you use your eyes to receive what is out there. Too often we strain the eyes when we try to take in too much. Or we avoid seeing by blocking what is out there. Observe your style of looking. Do not judge. Create new possibilities by staying present through your eyes. See how it feels.

You can now begin helping yourself reclaim your natural right to see without glasses. Enjoy!

Dr. Roberto Kaplan
Vienna, Austria

How to Use This Book

Seeing Without Glasses: A Step-by-Step Approach to Improving Eyesight Naturally is divided into four parts.

Part 1 deals with fitness of the eye at a physical level. It assesses the components of vision-fitness, examines environmental and other aspects of our culture that play a role in the loss of vision-fitness, helps you to learn how your eyes—aided by special vision-fitness lenses—can provide feedback to alert you to aspects of your lifestyle that may be affecting your seeing, and introduces you to exercises designed to enhance the performance of the individual structures of your eyes.

Part 2 explores the idea that fluctuations in vision-fitness occur as a normal variation of your daily living. It teaches you to recognize how your predominant visual style—being and seeing or doing and looking—affects the way you approach situations in your daily life. We investigate the behaviors associated with each visual style and describe techniques you can use to modify your behavior to fit changing life situations. Part Two also examines how the way you feed and exercise your body can affect the way you see, and it outlines guides for monitoring the effect of particular foods and levels of physical activity on your vision. Using these techniques, you can learn to nurture your body for maximum general physical fitness as well as vision-fitness.

Part 3 introduces the concept of the mind's eye and explains how the way you interpret events internally can have a bearing on your vision. It also illustrates why high-level vision-fitness depends on your right and left eyes participating harmoniously in what is called "whole-brain" processing, and it describes how you can achieve this healthy balance.

Part 4 gives you an opportunity to begin the *Seeing Without Glasses* program for improving your vision in three phases. It carefully takes you through all the phases step by step, explaining how to do the exercises, how to monitor biofeedback, and how to track your progress.

Each part of this book is self-contained, and I invite you to explore the depth and level of vision-fitness that suits your needs. Parts 1 through 3 will introduce you to the theory, research, and clinical evidence underlying the vision-fitness approach of *Seeing Without Glasses*. I recommend that you read all three parts at least once through to familiarize yourself with their language and concepts. Then use any of the ideas or exercises (vision games) that relate to your particular situation. Part 4 presents a deeper explanation of how to develop a vision-fitness program for yourself. The material is presented in such a way that, depending on your needs, you might use any or all of the elements of the program. At certain times you may desire to apply nutritional aspects to your life, while later, wearing an eye patch may look like fun. You may select certain vision games and aerobic or movement exercises, or you might commit to the whole program. Whatever your level of involvement, you will improve your vision. You can repeat any of the processes whenever you feel the need.

I often remind my patients and myself that helping your eyes and vision is a journey. Sometimes you may need a rest stop. At other times you will wish to move full steam ahead. Whichever path you follow, perform with great attention to quality!

Introduction

In our Western culture, having 20/20 vision signifies an ideal level of normalcy that is based on a perception which has been perpetuated by the vision-care industry. If you can see a one-inch letter at a distance of 20 feet, then your vision is considered "normal." Whether the diagnosis comes from a school nurse, your eye doctor, or your family physician, when you hear 20/20, you breathe a sigh of relief. If you wear eyeglasses or contacts, they artificially induce 20/20, and you're thankful for that. You are probably reading this book to find out how you can maintain 20/20 vision or how you can reach it without eyeglasses.

First, you must understand that in our culture a state of clear vision is the exception rather than the rule. Why is it that in the United States more than 100 million people are nearsighted (have difficulty seeing small detail at a distance) and at least six out of ten rely on artificial devices in order to see clearly? Why are so many people being diagnosed with potentially life-threatening eye diseases, such as macular degeneration, cataracts, glaucoma, and detachments, and yet no additional help beyond medications and surgery is being offered? Their choices are severely limited in spite of an abundance of complementary procedures, known and somewhat available, which could help individuals if they were willing to learn how to implement these self-help tools.

Even if you have 20/20 vision and don't need to wear corrective devices, you are likely among the growing number of people who are experiencing increasing degrees of eyestrain. Symptoms including burning, itching, blurriness, tearing, reduced comprehension with sustained reading, and aching usually coincide with a drop in visual efficiency. They can be an indication that your ability for your eyes to be directed by your brain is diminishing. Fortunately, you can correct the problem by learning a series of skills that can be practiced and perfected in much the same way you would learn to play a musical instrument. The exercises are simple, and you will notice the results immediately.

Seeing Without Glasses teaches you new ways to enhance your vision performance and thus complement your vision-care program with your eye doctor. This approach incorporates techniques developed by the science of eye refraction, diagnosis, and treatment of eye diseases, the technology of lens prescription, vision therapy, and the use of complementary methods. These methods acknowledge the healing power of vitamins, minerals, and herbs and emphasize your role in the healing process. The primary purpose of this book is to inspire you to take charge of the well-being of your own eyes and vision and to teach you how best to use your eye doctor as a support person.

The directions outlined in this book are based on one key premise: Just as you can develop your physical fitness, you can also improve the fitness of your eyes—the way they work together, their stamina, and their interaction with your brain. Your eye doctor has probably made a diagnosis and treatment predictions based on a standard Western model. *Seeing Without Glasses* presents a bridge between the technology of Western medical science and the wisdom of intuitive healing. By adding this complementary approach, you are empowered to change your doctor's prognosis.

Seeing Without Glasses presents an opportunity to look beyond what you accept as normal, to open up the reality that improving vision-fitness is possible.

You may be wondering if I am suggesting that you immediately throw away your eyeglasses or contacts. No. I suggest that your eye devices, like weights, running shoes, or a tennis racquet, can be utilized as therapeutic tools. When the prescription is appropriately designed, it will help your eyes and your brain relearn how to work as a team.

As your vision-fitness increases, you will continue to develop a new therapeutic relationship with your glasses. Even if you don't currently use eye devices, you'll notice an increased ability to use your eyes for tasks like reading, fine detail work, computer work, judging distances, and sports.

By better understanding how your eyes work and can develop or lose vision-fitness, you'll become an active participant in their care. Just as your car lets you know when you need gas, an oil change, or service, you'll learn to recognize when your eyes are calling for a rest break or a vision-fitness exercise.

Your eyes are constantly giving you feedback. The vision-fitness program laid out in this book will teach you to interpret and be sensitive to what your eyes are telling you. Whether you wear glasses, have an eye disease, or have basic symptoms of blurry vision or tired eyes, there is a subtle message being conveyed through your eyes. When my patients discover this hidden communication, their eyes almost always begin to feel healthier and their vision gets sharper.

Seeing Without Glasses looks to the future in vision care, a future that will involve you as an active participant in the prevention of eye problems and the maintenance of high-level vision-fitness. This doesn't mean that your eye doctor will become obsolete. Rather, the role of your optometrist or ophthalmologist will be that of teacher, facilitator, or guide in your quest for optimum vision-fitness.

Vision-fitness programs are being incorporated into schools so that children can protect and strengthen their vision through the use of special exercises. Specialized applications of vision therapy are even being used to help people with learning and reading difficulties. People who have been labeled dyslexic—who face reading challenges such as letter and word reversals, transpositions, and substitutions—are using vision-fitness and therapy to reduce the dyslexic behaviors.

Even if you don't have a specific vision problem, using the vision-fitness approach will improve the quality of your work life. In fact, vision-fitness techniques are now being used in employee-wellness programs to help offset the high incidence of eyestrain associated with the modern workplace populated by computers and other electronic gadgetry. And by practicing these vision-fitness techniques, you will also gain insight into the way the eyes work and the process of vision.

Perhaps you are wondering why this thinking isn't more commonplace. Why has your past vision care not included prevention and improvement? Why is this form of vision care limited to a few thousand optometrists who specialize in behavioral vision therapy?

There are many answers to these questions. I will attempt to give you a succinct overview by describing my own perspective. In my experience as a professor in two professional schools of optometry in Texas and Oregon, I observed the training of doctors of optometry. They are primarily taught that treatment of vision-fitness requires the application of eyeglasses or contacts. This traditional viewpoint asserts that if your eyes are defective, you need a "corrective" device to compensate for the imperfection. It would stand to reason that "corrective" tools like lenses would eventually be removed once the therapy is completed. This, however, is not the case. Lens prescriptions typically become stronger over time, which leads to greater and greater dependency on the corrective devices, which is as insidious in its own way as a dependency on sugar, drugs, or alcohol.

I was a victim of that thinking when I was being trained as an eye doctor. I really believed that recommending full-strength lens prescriptions for my patients would help their eyes to "get better." After working with thousands of patients as an optometrist, I realized that I was actually contributing to their vision loss.

What follows in the upcoming pages is a summary of how I complement regular vision programs with concrete help. This integration goes beyond the palliative effects of strong eyeglasses. Vision-fitness requires you to take responsibility for your vision, using vision games that are suited to your needs and condition. The vision games stimulate or relax your eyes and your mind in order to restore their natural resilience and power. You are your own best teacher, and it is up to you to incorporate these practices into your daily life. Be careful not to fall prey to the notion that the exercises are fixing something that is faulty. Your loss of vision-fitness is simply telling you about the abuse, strain, and distress of your eyes and giving you an opportunity to make a change for the better.

Using the information in this book, you can improve your vision using the same techniques I use myself. I was able to stop wearing glasses entirely and to reduce the presence of double vision almost 95 percent. Others have reduced their need to wear glasses by between 40 and 100 percent. Some patients have regenerated parts of their eye tissue even though their eye doctor had emphatically stated that no cure was possible. Don't give up hope. Seek a second opinion. Practice the techniques in this book. Feel free to contact me personally. I can conduct a consultation by long-distance telephone/fax or audiotape in order to create a personalized approach for your use of *Seeing Without Glasses*. Enjoy your discoveries!

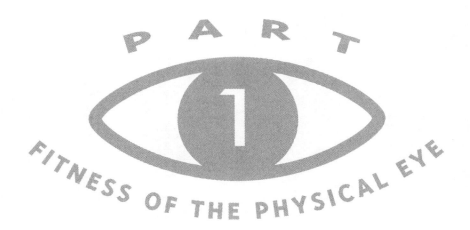

PART 1

1

FITNESS OF THE PHYSICAL EYE

Chapter 1

What Is Vision-Fitness?

Your eyes, for their size, have a greater blood and nerve supply than most of the other organ systems in the body, and there is a strong relationship between the brain and the fitness of the eyes. Approximately 49 percent of the brain's cranial nerves, which directly feed the body's nervous system, are just for the eyes.

In the book *Total Fitness*, authors Morehouse and Gross define fitness as the ability to meet the demands of one's environment. Vision-fitness has to do with the clarity of your seeing, the degree of partnership between your two eyes, and making sense of what you see in your environment. We can speak of natural, or "naked," vision-fitness (without corrective devices) as well as the degree of vision-fitness induced by eyeglasses or contact lenses.

Clarity of Seeing

Some of you may have observed or may have been told that your vision is not 20/20. This loss of seeing, or blurred vision, can be considered a drop in vision-fitness.

Even if you naturally have 20/20 vision, you might experience eyestrain, burning or itching eyes, double vision, fatigue, loss of comprehension, or poor attention span. These symptoms or behaviors are indicative of poor visual fitness or stamina. (In some cases, disease of the eyes produces a loss of natural vision-fitness. This disease aspect will be discussed in a later chapter.)

If you have lost your ability to see clearly at the reading distance, this is yet another loss of vision-fitness. In this case the focusing/lens system of your eyes is losing its natural ability or fitness to perform. While most eye doctors view this loss as a consequence of natural aging, I have had the opportunity to see patients who prolong their ability to focus clearly and avoid the total loss of focusing by improving their vision-fitness.

Mary, age fifty-five, was farsighted and was wearing recently prescribed bifocals, which provide one focus for near and one for far distances. After one month of using the vision-fitness techniques outlined in this book, Mary was able to wear single-vision reading glasses equivalent in power to those she had when she was in her early forties. Mary did not throw away her eyeglasses. What she did was restore thirteen years of vision-fitness.

You can also use the vision-fitness approach if you're nearsighted and/or have astigmatism. Nearsightedness means that you are unable to see distant objects clearly. Astigmatism usually refers to a cornea that has unequal curvature in the different meridians. As a result, you have to focus different amounts and your vision can be affected by blur, double vision, straining, and even headaches.

Linda had nearsightedness and astigmatism for over twenty-five years. She was required to wear corrective lenses for driving. Linda began to improve her vision-fitness, and within six months from the time she began to utilize the concepts and techniques from this book, she was able to pass the driver's eye test. For the first time in nineteen years of driving, Linda was able to drive legally without corrective lenses. At the age of thirty-six, Linda was able to see as she had when she was seventeen. She restored her vision without a need for eyeglasses or contacts.

The Partnership of Your Eyes

For those who need eyeglasses or contacts, 95 percent of the time eye doctors prescribe a full-strength prescription for 20/20. But in my research on stress and two-eyedness, I have found that in 75 percent of cases, full-strength lens prescriptions for nearsightedness and astigmatism produce distress (unmanageable stress) related to the way patients use their eyes together.

Your doctor will probably determine your lens prescription by testing each eye separately, assuming that this "single-eye-tested" prescription will serve you in a "two-eyed-looking" world. My clinical research, however, has demonstrated that the single-eye-tested prescriptions tend to be too strong, and I believe that this ultimately plays a role in diminishing vision-fitness.

I have tested patients with both their eyes open for many years, and I have discovered that lens prescriptions determined by single-eye exams are often too strong. Reducing the power of the corrective lenses helps the eyes work better together, thereby increasing overall vision-fitness and minimizing eyestrain and fatigue.

What about eye partnership in persons who do not wear corrective lenses? A large percentage of people who have 20/20 vision have difficulty with tasks involving close work. Your eyes are biologically unsuited for the kinds of close work you demand of them. Your eyes are designed for three-dimensional, fast-moving, and multifocal viewing. But computer screens, books, newspapers, and other detailed objects make your eyes focus at one distance in two dimensions only. Consequently, reading for long periods, looking at a computer screen, sewing, and other near-distance work can produce varying intensities of eyestrain. Since these symptoms are unrelated to clarity, I find the difficulty, in 70 percent of cases, to be in how the eyes work together as a team. Fortunately, vision-fitness exercises can help you develop greater two-eyed fitness.

Making Sense of What You See

You may be able to hit a fast-moving ball, read words and sentences, and observe data on a computer screen without difficulty. But when you have to process information at higher degrees of understanding, you tend to make less sense of what you are seeing. For example, even if you have 20/20 vision, you may find that after reading for a while, your mind wanders, and you get sleepy, daydream, or become bored. Maybe you can enter data into a computer, but you find that following logical patterns of thought, retrieving sequenced data consistently, or tracking fast-moving objects for long periods of time causes eye fatigue.

People who fall into this category—having good clarity but some difficulty interpreting what they see—tend to be a little farsighted. It's as if their eyes are designed for far looking. On the other hand, those who wear glasses and contacts for nearsightedness tend to be good readers and excellent students because their eyes are well adapted for reading.

All three aspects of vision-fitness decrease over time. It's as if our eyes run out of gas as we age. Even so, vision-fitness, like body fitness, can be improved. Your eye muscles can be exercised. The nerve connection from the brain to your eyes can be stimulated. Blood flow to your eyes can be increased. The vision-fitness exercises in this book will teach you to maximize your vision and to increase your overall feeling of well-being.

How Fit Is Your Vision?

From case histories and clinical research we find that certain behaviors are related to vision-fitness. The following questionnaire will help you identify particular behaviors that apply to your vision-fitness.* Indicate on a scale from zero to ten how difficult these activities are for you.

If you gave yourself a score of five or higher on an item, your ability to perform that activity could be improved by better vision-fitness.

---

*Some questions were modified from *Eye Power* (Alfred A. Knopf, Inc.). Copyright © 1979 by Ann and Townsend Hoopes.

Vision-Fitness Questionnaire

	No	Yes	Unbearable
1. Do you have difficulty in completing a near-distance assignment (e.g., reading, writing a letter, or studying)?	0 1 2 3 4 5 6 7 8 9 10		
2. Do you experience difficulty when shifting from one activity to another (e.g., working on a project and then going to cook)?	0 1 2 3 4 5 6 7 8 9 10		
3. Do you find playing and enjoying tennis, basketball, or any other game involving fast-moving balls and players difficult?	0 1 2 3 4 5 6 7 8 9 10		
4. Is your reading speed slow (200 words per minute or less), or have you noticed a drop in your reading speed?	0 1 2 3 4 5 6 7 8 9 10		
5. Do you have difficulty reading maps or visualizing geometry?	0 1 2 3 4 5 6 7 8 9 10		
6. Do you have difficulty visualizing something you're reading about or imagining "as if" situations (e.g., trying to imagine the sun shining on a rainy day)?	0 1 2 3 4 5 6 7 8 9 10		
7. Have you experienced difficulty with hidden-word games, losing your sense of direction, or keeping your place while following directions or reading?	0 1 2 3 4 5 6 7 8 9 10		
8. Is it hard for you to read for pleasure?	0 1 2 3 4 5 6 7 8 9 10		
9. Do you have difficulty concentrating on concurrent events (e.g., following a lecture while taking notes)?	0 1 2 3 4 5 6 7 8 9 10		
10. Does your stomach bother you when you read in the back seat of a car?	0 1 2 3 4 5 6 7 8 9 10		
11. Is it a challenge for you to organize your visual and mental capacities to read and write effectively (e.g., following an author's point of view or writing a short story)?	0 1 2 3 4 5 6 7 8 9 10		

(continued on next page)

	No	Yes	Unbearable
Vision-Fitness Questionnaire, cont'd.			

	No	Yes	Unbearable
12. Are you disappointed by your performance in reading and writing (see no. 11)?	0 1 2 3 4 5 6 7 8 9 10		
13. Is it hard for you to accurately recall or reproduce a drawn, written, or visual presentation of what you've seen (e.g., observing a scene and then listing what you saw without rechecking)?	0 1 2 3 4 5 6 7 8 9 10		
14. Is it hard for you to solve practical or theoretical problems without using paper and a pen or pencil?	0 1 2 3 4 5 6 7 8 9 10		
15. Is your visual attention poorer when there is movement, or does the horizon appear to move up and down when you walk?	0 1 2 3 4 5 6 7 8 9 10		
16. Do you find it awkward to judge where objects are located (e.g., judging the distance when you reach out to find something)?	0 1 2 3 4 5 6 7 8 9 10		
17. Do you often misjudge an object's true position (see no. 16)?	0 1 2 3 4 5 6 7 8 9 10		
18. Are you bothered by crowds in theaters, department stores, or shopping centers?	0 1 2 3 4 5 6 7 8 9 10		
19. Do you have difficulty tracking (following) an object moving laterally or vertically?	0 1 2 3 4 5 6 7 8 9 10		

Having read this far, you should now be better prepared to participate as an intelligent consumer in your vision-care program. Armed with questions and new insight into your vision-fitness, you can be ready to request the kind of vision care you desire. Find a vision-fitness-oriented optometrist or ophthalmologist who will work with you.

Chapter 2

Loss of Vision-Fitness

Less than 10 percent of the population is born with blurred vision, upset binocularity (two-eyedness), or diseased eyes. But by young adulthood, a disturbing 60 percent of the remaining 90 percent have nearsightedness, farsightedness, astigmatism, crossed or wall eyes, or ocular-disease conditions. This provocative statistic clearly demonstrates that we as a culture are slowly losing our natural vision-fitness.

From the time we are born until adulthood, our interaction with our environment leads to a drop in vision-fitness. In interviewing thousands of patients, I determined some of the environmental and other factors that play a part in the evolution and development of eye and vision problems (these are not ranked in any order):

- Inappropriate eating patterns, such as excessive intake of simple carbo-hydrates and over-refined foods, and eating while emotionally upset

- Going to school

- Poor reading habits

- Air, water, and food pollutants (chemicals, preservatives, etc.)

- Excessive sugar consumption

- Too little exposure to sunlight

- Poorly designed workplaces

- Achievement-oriented schooling and sports

- Lack of physical exercise

- Breakup of the traditional family model

- Divorce

- Frequent moves

- Excessive viewing of television

- Poorly monitored use of computers

- Denial and addictive patterns of behavior

If you ever have a chance to spend time around aboriginal people, especially in non-industrialized countries, notice how their eyes move around. They rapidly shift their focus from close to distant objects. Their eyes scan left to right, up and down, and diagonally, stretching the muscles.

The human eye is designed to move, stretch, and focus at far distances. The eyes are designed for hunting, gathering berries, growing crops, and farming. Industrialized culture, however, has developed technology that requires your natural vision-fitness to be modified. Your eyes must adjust to long hours sitting at a desk, looking at a terminal screen, typing, reviewing computer-printout sheets, reading books, working with fine eye-hand coordination, and the myriad of academic and job-related tasks you demand of your eyes. Your eyes are also forced to adjust to artificial fluorescent lighting, filtered air conditioning and heating, and the bombardment of particles from synthetic carpeting, desks, chairs, paper, inks, and paints. This is a far cry from the green forests, lushly carpeted grasslands, and pristine mountaintops of your counterparts living in nature.

Moreover, you also encounter the challenges of quotas, deadlines, dealing with co-workers, and financial budgeting. All these stressors can ultimately affect the fitness of your eyes. You may notice that on the days when you are more relaxed, your ability to use your eyes efficiently is greater.

These environmental changes haven't happened overnight. There has been an insidious slow movement to the point where over 100 million people in the United States now require eyeglasses or contacts for nearsightedness. Your brain and eyes have had to adjust from far looking to concentrating on schoolwork and office tasks. Nearsightedness is a perfect adaptation. You maintain high vision-fitness up close at the expense of clarity at intermediate or far distances.

Chapter 1 mentioned the distress that can be brought about by looking through full-strength eyeglass or contact-lens prescriptions. The strength of the distance-viewing prescription may be too strong for close work. Seventy percent of the time, a lens prescription is designed for looking at a far distance, which produces distress while looking at a closer distance. It's not so much that things look blurry up close, but you experience discomfort, a feeling of tiredness, or even sleepiness while reading, doing computer work, and other close-distance looking. This may also occur if you have 20/20 vision without lenses.

What may be happening is that your eyes are giving you feedback that you are experiencing a drop in vision-fitness. Over time, your eyes may no longer be able to cooperate as partners. Your brain, in desperation, may finally decide to shut off one of the images.

Typically, if you receive this kind of feedback, you'll think that there's something "wrong." You may rationalize that you're tired. You may feel that your eyes are getting weak or that you need a stronger lens prescription. *Seeing Without Glasses* presents another choice. You can view this symptom as you would a red warning light in your car and take steps to restore your vision-fitness.

What should you do if you receive feedback that your vision-fitness is dropping? One of the first signs of distress in the body is holding one's breath, or shallow breathing. Shallow breathing can deprive the eyes of essential nutrients, as they are situated far from the heart and lungs. Your vision may appear blurry or gray. And more than likely you'll be staring—maybe even with your head thrust a little forward. To see the best example of this, watch the people next to you at the stoplight at 5:00 P.M. on a weekday. Are they staring aimlessly into space, not blinking?

Check your breathing. Is it shallow? Breathe deeply. Hear the sounds. Feel your chest and stomach moving. Blink your eyelids. Check your body posture. It's like pulling into a service station and checking the water level, oil level, and tire pressure for your car.

As more people suffer vision loss as a result of eyestrain in their offices and at home, it is more important than ever to take steps to improve vision-fitness. You could ignore the reality of vision-fitness loss and become solely reliant on artificial devices, or just as you may be cultivating your body fitness and nutritional well-being, you can begin to improve and maintain your vision-fitness. Begin protecting your vision by being aware of when your vision-fitness decreases.

Chapter 3

The Eyes As a
Biofeedback Mechanism

In Western cultures, the eyes are the point of focus during most forms of interpersonal communication. Your eyes are indeed "the window to your soul." They reveal an extraordinary degree of non-verbal communication.

If you are aware of your eyes, you will notice that they provide feedback about the effects of many variables in your life. You may recall from the previous chapter that many factors in your internal (mental and emotional) and external environments can lead to a drop in vision-fitness. The food you eat, the way you exercise, the way you relate to others, and satisfaction or upsets in relationships can all cause fluctuations in the quality of your vision.

The loss of vision-fitness takes place over time. You do not become nearsighted, farsighted, or develop astigmatism overnight. An astute, developmentally interested optometrist can monitor the stages of vision-fitness loss. And in the same way, as you redevelop fitness in your seeing, the changes can be measured physically in the eye.

Hearing What Your Eyes Are Saying

Let's go a little deeper into this concept of how your eyes can act as a biofeedback mechanism. First, let's review what 20/20 eyesight means. The 20/20 refers to the measurement of how well you see. If you can see a one-inch letter at a distance of 20 feet, your doctor will give you a rating of 20/20. On the other hand, if you can see the letter designed for 40 feet at 20 feet, your rating will be 20/40, and so on.

Most eye doctors determine the refraction (measurement of the eye prescription) needed to provide you with 100 percent ability to perform visual discrimination at 20 feet—a standard set many years ago.

This standard course of treatment is far from ideal. Years ago, many of my patients began asking me if there was any way they could improve their eyesight naturally. They were concerned that each time they visited me, I would pass on the news that their prescription needed to be stronger.

In response, I began to experiment, reducing the power of patients' lens prescriptions. After a number of research trials, the optimum vision-fitness level seemed to be around 83.6 percent. If the vision clarity was less than 83.6 percent, the world appeared too blurry and patients' frustration level was too high, thus defeating their natural seeing capabilities. If their vision was clearer than 83.6 percent, there was not enough blur to encourage the patients to develop their vision-fitness. This meant that I would measure the patient for 20/40. If the patient was nearsighted and/or had astigmatism, I reduced the power equally for the two conditions. For farsightedness, I used the far and/or near Eye-C charts (see chapter 12) and made similar reductions in power.

The overall response from the thousands of patients who took part in this ongoing experiment was that they loved their new vision-fitness prescriptions. Their looking appeared softer and generally produced a calming effect. When these patients looked at far distances, closer objects automatically became clearer. This meant that while looking at ten feet, their vision-fitness increased to 100 percent.

You might be asking the question, Why wear or use a lens prescription that does not completely correct your vision? Besides the behavioral advantages already mentioned, a reduced prescription allows you to teach your brain and your eyes to work more harmoniously as partners. If you wear a prescription that gives you 20/40 vision, or 83.6 percent vision-fitness, you can train your brain, eyes, and muscles to make up the other 16.4 percent, giving you 20/20 vision with this prescription.

This lens prescription can be called a vision-fitness type because while wearing the prescription (preferably in eyeglasses because of ease of removal), there will be times during the day when you will be able to monitor changes in vision-fitness. My patients have reported that their vision-fitness is affected by many elements of their lifestyles, including foods they eat, posture, aerobic exercise, level of stress on the job, reading patterns, working for extended periods at a computer, weather changes, and emotional fluctuations. (The way that some of these factors affect vision-fitness is discussed in chapters 6 through 9.)

Observing the fluctuation in the quality of your vision allows you to learn how to interpret the feedback your eyes provide. For example, if you notice that your vision-fitness drops as job stress increases, you can learn to take action to alleviate stress. Recall that by breathing deeply you can send extra oxygen and nutrients to the eyes to increase their function. Focusing to your nose (like crossing your eyes) and then looking off into the distance can also bring about a remarkable increase in vision-fitness. Over time, by employing vision-fitness exercises and making lifestyle changes as needed, you can stabilize your vision-fitness at 100 percent through the vision-fitness lenses. Then you can have your doctor order an even more reduced lens prescription and begin the process once again.

As you reduce the power in your lenses, your natural vision-fitness without lenses will also improve. You will be wearing lenses that are weaker, you will see more clearly without lenses, and you will be in control of how you use your glasses.

In the course of my clinical experiments comparing full-strength prescriptions with vision-fitness prescriptions, I have discovered that patients who wear full-strength prescriptions full time have less tolerance for visual stress than those wearing fitness prescriptions. Patients using full-strength prescriptions experience reduced depth perception and report that their lenses produce strain or fatigue after long-term use.

Thus, it seems that the brain "prefers" the 83.6 percent vision-fitness prescription, which gives the brain and the eyes a chance to be exercised. Just like the other muscles of the body, the brain and eyes respond well to being exercised. Imagine trying to exercise an injured arm while wearing a tight splint. Loosen the splint and there's more flexibility. The vision-fitness lens prescription is like a loosened splint. Looking through fitness lenses allows your eyes to get the exercise they need in order to get stronger.

Although vision-fitness is defined a little differently for people who already have 20/20 vision, they too can use the feedback they get from their eyes to increase productivity and to decrease fatigue and strain. For example, recall how you feel after reading for extended periods. Does your comprehension drop? Does your mind wander? Do you become sleepy? Even if you have 20/20 vision, your vision-fitness for memory retention and recall of details may be lower than that of someone who has 20/50 vision.

If you experience a loss of comprehension or have trouble paying attention even though you have 20/20 vision, it probably means that the function of your eye muscles and the accuracy of input to the brain from the eyes needs to be enhanced. Often persons with natural 20/20 vision have an impaired ability to coordinate their eyes. You might experience fatigue after a lot of close work, eyestrain or intermittent blurring while working at a computer screen, burning eyes after reading, or dry eyes while concentrating on any other near-distance task as a result of the lack of coordination.

For some people, a specially designed near-distance lens can facilitate greater vision-fitness. It will not necessarily provide increased clarity, rather, a marked change in visual comfort. These lenses are called "stress-relieving lenses," or "focusing lenses." I strongly recommend that the lenses be used in conjunction with vision-fitness exercises so that you don't become addicted to the lenses. A good way to check your level of dependence is to see if near-distance material seems more blurry when you remove the lenses. If so, the lenses may be reducing your natural vision-fitness.

The purpose for wearing any of the lenses we've described above, then, is to help you see more clearly in the interim while you use special techniques to develop vision-fitness. Eyeglasses and contact lenses should be thought of as therapeutic devices that facilitate increased vision-fitness.

The following case studies further illustrate how reduced-power lenses combined with use of the biofeedback principle can help you improve your vision-fitness.

Steven, age twenty-four, began wearing reduced-power vision-fitness lenses. The following day he went with his friend George to play a game of racquetball. On entering the court, Steven casually glanced around through his new 20/40 eyeglasses and noticed that he could just barely make out the time on the wall clock. After forty minutes of racquetball, Steven once again glanced up at the clock as they were leaving the court. The time was perfectly clear (100 percent vision-fitness)—his vision-fitness had increased! Steven received clear feedback that aerobic exercise such as racquetball produces increased seeing for him.

Of course this called for a celebration, so Steven and George went out and had a few beers and hearty helpings of nachos, followed by a sugary dessert. As Steven looked around the restaurant, he noticed his vision-fitness dropping. Again, Steven received feedback—certain foods are undesirable. Steven could choose to avoid these foods or to exercise more vigorously after consuming these foods.

Anne, age thirty, is a computer programmer. She spends four to eight hours per day in front of a computer terminal. As an experiment, she placed an eye chart on the wall behind her monitor. The chart was about ten feet away, which meant that if she could see the twenty line, she had 20/40 vision-fitness. Each morning Anne checked her natural vision-fitness, monitoring the changes. She noticed that her vision-fitness dropped after about three hours of continuous work.

After consulting with me, Anne began to use vision-fitness techniques, such as focusing on the chart and stretching her eyes up and down while paying attention to her breathing. (For descriptions of these exercises, see chapter 12.) For Anne, breathing was one of the most important exercises, because whenever the task she was performing became complex, she literally held her breath. Anne also reported staring at the screen without blinking after a few hours of work. Employing the vision-fitness exercises, Anne was able to improve her vision-fitness to the point where the distressful symptoms were minimal. When she received feedback of distress, she employed the techniques to restore the fitness. Vision-fitness is like body fitness—once you begin to achieve fitness, you need to adopt a maintenance program.

Patients who have 20/20, or 100 percent vision-fitness, also report fluctuations in their clear seeing when engaged in reading, sewing, crocheting, computer programming, painting, and other near-distance activities. Even if you don't require corrective lenses, you can still use visual feedback to maintain good vision.

Whenever you notice that your vision is blurry, strained, or distorted, take time out from the activity to breathe deeply, focus your attention and your eyes to a different distance, stretch your body muscles, yawn, and blink your eyes. These are easy, basic techniques for maintaining high levels of vision-fitness.

Your emotional and mental states of mind can also affect your vision-fitness. It seems to me that adults—young and old—laugh less than they used to. What do you think will happen to your seeing if you are sad or despondent? Smiling, laughing, and being joyous will allow you to increase your vision-fitness.

Wear your vision-fitness lenses, focus more gently, and smile, and your whole body and state of being will feel more relaxed.

Summary

- Sit down and practice being still. Close your eyes in order to deepen your sense of peacefulness. Focus on your breathing and direct your attention to your heart.

- Blink every three to five seconds.

- Direct your breath into the inner heart chamber. Continue breathing until you feel your heart opening more and more. You will probably experience a calm, warm feeling.

- Remember that your heart represents compassion, kindness, and love.

- Open your eyes, and using your new awareness, look around with love.

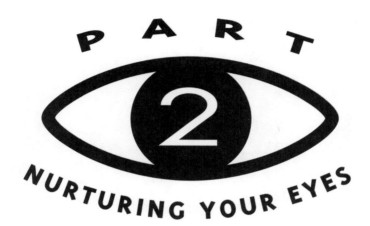

PART

2

NURTURING YOUR EYES

Chapter 4

Exercising the Muscles of the Eyes

To fully utilize the vision-fitness program in this book, it is helpful to have some basic knowledge about the structures of the eye and how they work. This chapter will take you on a journey through the parts of the eye, explaining their purpose, how they work, and strategies that can be incorporated to enhance their fitness. Learning to picture the anatomy of the eye will help you to achieve the best results from the vision-fitness exercises in this and other chapters.

The Cornea

The cornea is the shiny, curved part of the outside of the eye. It covers the iris (the pigmented part). The cornea controls 80 percent of the refracting power of the eye. The cornea derives its nutrients from tears, which also act as a lubricant. Tear fluid is distributed over the cornea when you blink. The types of activities to which you subject your eyes determine how much you blink. For example, looking at a computer screen, reading, watching television, doing near-distance work, and driving a car can lead to staring, which slows your rate of blinking, resulting in dry eyes. Wearing contact lenses can also interfere with the optimum blink rate, which is about once every three seconds. The lids treat the contact lens as a foreign body, and your brain sends a message to the lids to blink less. When you do not blink often enough, your eyes do not receive adequate nutrients or moisture. Consequently, you might experience burning, itching, gritty, heavy, or watery eyes. This is feedback—a reminder to blink. Blinking every three seconds is one of the first ways to enhance your vision-fitness.

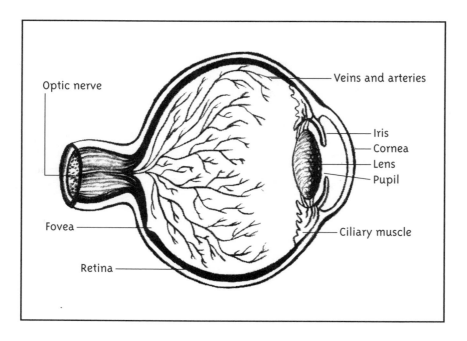

The Iris and the Pupil

The iris is the colored membrane between the cornea and the lens. The muscle of the iris is stimulated by the absence or presence of light. When there's plenty of light, the muscle contracts, causing the pupil (the black aperture in the center of the iris) to get smaller. In the dark, the muscle relaxes and the pupil gets larger. In this way, the iris regulates the amount of light entering the eye.

The way in which the iris regulates the amount of light entering the eye is enhanced by full-spectrum sunlight. There is a growing body of evidence that the light which enters your eyes, especially natural sunlight, plays an important role in balancing your nervous system. During a typical day, you use incandescent or fluorescent light sources, and you look through windows, car windshields, eyeglasses, and contacts, which absorb some of the near-ultraviolet rays of sunlight. The loss of natural, or full-spectrum, light means that you are not exposed to enough near-ultraviolet light rays, and your nervous system must compensate. This compensation disturbs the natural balance of the body and ultimately of the organ structures, including the eyes.

John Ott, author of *Light, Radiation and You*, has written that the presence of full-spectrum light permits maximum narrowing of the pupil. When devices that absorb the near-ultraviolet are worn, he says, a larger pupil is measured. For many years my colleague Dr. Raymond Gottlieb and I have hypothesized that having enlarged pupils on a chronic basis may predispose certain persons to glaucoma (a buildup in pressure behind the eye). In fact, for patients who have been diagnosed as having glaucoma, a medication that reduces the pupil size is routinely prescribed. The wider the pupil, the more likely that pressure will build up behind the eye and block the flow of fluids. Sunlight can naturally create the same result as medication. Some of my patients with "thin-angle" glaucoma have been able to reduce their medication as their vision-fitness developed under the supervision of their ophthalmologist. It is imperative that you consult with your ophthalmologist before reducing your medication.

I suggest spending about twenty minutes per day outside with your head toward the sun and your eyes closed. Feel the warmth on your face. Imagine a packet of warm energy entering your body through your closed eyelids and striking the iris. Feel the pupil closing. Visualize how small it is. Blink and let the pupil get smaller when the light enters the eye. After the blink, visualize the pupil getting bigger.

Begin to move your chin slowly toward your left shoulder, and then toward your right shoulder, breathing deeply and occasionally blinking. If the sunlight is too intense, keep your eyes closed longer between blinks. If you notice a tendency to close one eye more than the other in sunlight, this may further confirm a lack of coordination between your eyes. This exercise will be described in more detail in chapter 12.

You might also want to see if you can reduce your need to wear sunglasses. If you ski, or if for occupational reasons you need to wear sunglasses, obtain a polaroid, a neutral gray tint, or a Rayban G15 tint. Your sight is worth the cost of a high-quality lens that you can be sure will absorb the undesirable short-ultraviolet frequency of light. If you are dependent on artificial light, choose full-spectrum fluorescent tubes or daylight-blue color-corrected full-spectrum incandescent bulbs. (See Vision-Improvement Programs and Services.)

The Lens and the Ciliary Muscle

The lens is a transparent convex structure that focuses the light entering through the pupil to form an image on the retina. The ciliary muscle governs the focusing of the eye by changing the shape of the lens. This "focusing" muscle is considered an involuntary muscle, that is, a muscle which you cannot consciously control. This means that if you overfocus, your ciliary muscle can become cramped and sluggish, which may cause your vision to appear blurry. You may also notice that it takes longer than usual to focus.

Stimulation of the ciliary muscle produces more power in the focusing ability of the lens, which enables you to focus on small details at closer distances, as when reading, sewing, crocheting, doing computer work, finding numbers in the phone book, and so on.

There are several things you can do to help maintain focusing fitness:

• Glance up at a far object and bring it quickly into focus every few minutes.

- Hold your thumb about six inches from your eyes. Focus on your thumbnail, then look off into the distance, and then focus back onto your thumb.

- Remember to breathe regularly when you are doing near-distance tasks.

- When you drive, "zoom" your focus to different objects—for example, the rear-view mirror, dashboard, license plate of the car in front of you, window, and then side mirror.

- While on the phone, focus on the receiver, objects on your desk, out the window, back to your pen, and so on.

Keep your eyes moving, focusing alternately on different distances, and your focusing muscles will become flexible and fit.

The Retina and the Fovea

The retina is the light-sensitive membrane lining the back of the eye. Light energy striking the retina is converted into chemical signals that carry information to the brain via the optic nerve. The retina serves to detect movement in one's peripheral (side) vision and to permit night vision.

The most acute visual perception takes place at a small area near the center of the retina called the fovea centralis. When the entering rays of light all focus clearly on the fovea, you see 20/20.

You must be careful not to strain your eyes as a result of trying to see clearly. Avoid staring at one place for an extended period. Let your eyes dance and move. Staring leads to an overstimulation of the fovea and to possible cramping of the focusing muscle, which, in turn, can result in less effective functioning of the retina, which means you'll miss some objects in your peripheral vision. When you are too foveal (focused), your vision-fitness percentage decreases. Simply put, you notice less in your environment. It's almost like being too self-focused.

The solution is to emulate the way indigenous people vigilantly scan their environment. Keep the eyes moving so that the fovea is constantly receiving new stimulation. Blink and breathe.

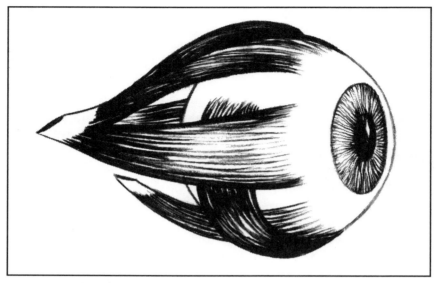

The Outside Muscles of the Eye

Each eye has six muscles surrounding the eyeball. The eyes can move up, down, left, right, inward, and outward, always paralleling each other. The muscles are attached to the sclera (the white of the eye). Your ability to coordinate the movement of these muscles greatly determines your level of vision-fitness.

In order to preserve the fitness of these muscles, you must exercise them just as you would any other muscle group, starting with a warm-up. Seat yourself comfortably, with your hands supported and both feet firmly on the ground. Your eyes may be either open or closed. Take a few deep breaths. When you are ready, stretch your eyes as high as they can go without straining while you inhale. Hold the breath, and when you are ready to exhale, stretch the muscles into the extreme downward position and breathe out. Repeat the up-and-down movement for three breaths. Next, stretch to the right. Then stretch up to the right and down to the left, and finally, up to the left and down to the right. If you feel any residual tension in the muscles, extend the breath slightly and reduce the degree of stretching. Avoid straining or extreme stretching. Remember, vision-fitness develops while exercising in a relaxed way. As with any fitness procedure, do a "cooling-off" exercise. Rub your hands together until your palms are warm, then gently cover your closed eyes with the palms of your hands. Overlap the fingers above the bridge of your nose to create as much darkness as possible. Keep your eyes covered for a minute or two, counting between twenty and fifty breaths. Not only will you relax your eyes, but you'll probably experience quietness of the mind as well. This is like a meditation for the eyes.

When you remove your palms, you'll observe that colors are much brighter, you'll see more contrast, and you'll enjoy a wonderful, relaxed feeling in your eyes and brow muscles. Check to see if your vision-fitness percentage has changed.

Here's another useful exercise: Turn your eyes in, crossing them. (No, they won't get stuck, regardless of what your mother told you.) Attempt to look at the bridge of your nose. If you can't focus on your nose, try focusing on your thumb a few inches away from your face. Then slowly bring the thumb toward your nose and feel the eye muscles pulling in. These inner recti muscles are the turning-in muscles. This turning-in is vitally important for efficient and prolonged reading. If the inner recti don't coordinate well, the eyes will rely on the ciliary (focusing) muscles instead, which could result in a focusing-muscle spasm and blurring. There is a connection between the turning-in of the eyes and the ability to focus. Have someone check that your eyes are turning in equally. Breathe in as you move your thumb toward your nose. Breathe out as you zoom your focus to a far-away object. Make sure your shoulders and body muscles are relaxed.

Practice this fitness exercise for ten to twenty breaths every day. You can remove your eyeglasses for these fitness routines. If you're a contact lens wearer and can remove them, do so; otherwise, leave them in.

One further suggestion: Spend time studying the diagrams of the eye, and try to become familiar enough with them that you can visualize the eye structures with your eyes closed. When you stretch the eye muscles, or zoom back and forth, or do other eye exercises, blink and breathe, and visualize the particular portion of your eye's anatomy that's being stimulated. Picturing the part that is being trained will improve your performance and further enhance your overall vision-fitness.

It doesn't take much time out of your day to do these exercises, and your eyes are worth it. Your eyes serve you well. Love them, exercise them, and maintain their vision-fitness.

Vision-Fitness Exercises for Specific Eye Parts

Eye Anatomy	Vision-Fitness Exercise
Cornea	Blinking every three seconds
Iris muscles/Pupil	Using full-spectrum lighting; exposing closed eyes to sunlight and blinking
Lens/Ciliary muscle	Breathing; zooming (near/far focusing)
Retina/Fovea	Non-staring; moving the eyes frequently
Eye muscles	Eye-muscle stretching
Overall eye/ mind relaxation	Palming the eyes
Overall eye fitness	Visualizing the parts of the eye while exercising

Chapter 5

Being and Seeing or Doing and Looking

When I think about *being* and *doing*, and how these states relate to vision, I am reminded of the movie *The Gods Must Be Crazy*. One day while minding his own business (that is, while *being*), a Bushman in southern Africa is suddenly confronted with a Coca-Cola bottle that has been dropped from a small airplane flying above. This Coca-Cola bottle triggers a series of events that shifts the Bushman's state from *being* to *doing*. The Bushman's formerly peaceful lifestyle comes to be filled with anxiety and aggression, and it begins to move at a faster pace. As the bottle is investigated by the tribe members, social interaction among the Bushmen also changes.

The Bushman's way of life before the Coke bottle typifies *being*. Most forms of relaxation, such as aerobic exercise, meditation, biofeedback, yoga, tai chi, and Feldenkreis, produce a bodily state of being. This quiet, gentle, calm state is associated with *seeing*. When you are being, you aren't concentrating on thinking or understanding. Via your eyes, you are more connected to the world around you. Visually, you can think of being as seeing with the retina. You see everything, but you don't pay attention to any one particular detail.

Doing, on the other hand, is related to *looking*. Can you imagine being a Bushman and suddenly having to determine the meaning of a Coca-Cola bottle? The bottle brought up all kinds of questions for the Bushman. Where did it come from? Was it a sign that the gods were angry? The bottle affected the traditional social interactions of the Bushman tribe, as the members became competitive and began fighting for the bottle—more doing! Doing is associated with thinking, questioning, analyzing, and looking for details. Doing may be thought of as looking with the fovea of the eye.

In Western culture, the environmental stimulation of television, automobiles, busy downtowns, schedules, going to school, financial pressures, and being busy promotes a *doing* state. Scientific inquiry in medicine, mathematics, and other forms of research requires doing.

If you spend too much time looking (doing), you promote a more foveal point of view, which in turn promotes overfocusing. This overfocusing begins in the mind (mental focus) and later leads to overstraining of the ciliary muscle (eye focus). If you reach that stage, you'll become aware of a drop in vision-fitness, such as blurring, eye fatigue, double vision, or staring.

Visually speaking, your fovea is overused in our modern world. This is one of the reasons your natural vision-fitness decreases. When there's an imbalance between the being and doing activities in your life, an imbalance also occurs in the brain. The vision-fitness approach calls for you to become aware of those times when you feel an imbalance between your being and doing as well as your seeing and looking.

Let's use the example of reading a book. You have eaten dinner and feel perfectly relaxed. You're sitting in your favorite chair, and the lighting is good. After about thirty minutes you catch yourself bringing the book closer to your eyes. Over time the distance between the book and your eyes decreases to six or eight inches. You also feel a little tension in your neck. What started off as a balanced being/doing activity became a doing task. The unconscious staring and "hard" focusing of the ciliary muscle produced a shift in energy flow from the brain. The reduced reading distance and neck tension were feedback from your body and eyes that your mind and eye muscles had become tense.

Other situations in which this can occur include watching television, working at a computer terminal, sewing, and similar near-distance work. Notice if your legs become tired or tense. Are your legs crossed? Are you frowning or squinting your eyes? After these kinds of activities, do your eyes feel heavy or ache? The classic indicators of movement from a being to a doing state are staring, shallow breathing, and non-blinking. Periodically check your posture, your breathing, your blinking, and your working distance.

What Is Your Visual Style?

The balanced being/doing concept, as it relates to vision-fitness, is associated with your visual style. You have acquired ways of looking at—or alternatively, seeing—situations in your life. The following exercise will help you determine your visual style. Do you favor seeing or looking? Circle the behaviors that apply to you.*

Being and Seeing Visual Style

- Scores better in reading than in math

- Tendency to lose place when reading or writing ideas

- Not precise with language or ideas

- Distractable, impulsive, fast but imprecise when performing detailed tasks

- Tendency for mind to drift, daydream, or "space out"

- Tendency to work from the general to the specific

*Some of these behaviors were shared by optometrist Dr. Richard Kavner through personal correspondence.

- More difficulty driving in the evening than in the morning

- Difficulty maintaining attention in detailed tasks

- Inability to sustain near-distance work; tendency to get sleepy

- Difficulty concentrating on continuing events, such as a lecture

- Tired to the point of irritability when getting home from work

Doing and Looking Visual Style

- Not always aware of the overall picture or the end result of an action

- Tendency to get caught up in projects and details

- Tendency to be precise and slow in tasks requiring a broad understanding

- Difficulty shifting attention from task to task, idea to idea

- Feel that you must finish the present task before starting another

- Difficulty pulling out into traffic

- Dislike ambiguity (situations involving contradictions)

- People say you tend to be too logical and analytical

- Give the impression of being a "know-it-all"

- Tendency not to notice things outside your immediate field of vision

Count the number of behaviors that you have circled for each of the two categories. Optimally, there should be an equal number for each style. If this is not so, which behaviors would you like to acquire or eliminate? Become aware of situations in your life that involve those desirable or undesirable behaviors. For example, if you find yourself rushing through a project and making careless mistakes, are you not focusing, that is, not doing enough? If so, how would you prefer to be performing at that moment? Find the vision-fitness exercise—most likely zooming, breathing, crossing your eyes, or palming—that will restore the balance between seeing and looking.

To further appreciate this balanced being/doing and seeing/looking concept, some understanding of the brain will be helpful. The brain has two hemispheres. In most people, the left brain performs the mathematical, speech, logical, analytical, linear, and rhythmical functions. The right brain, for most people, is the seat of creative, artistic, musical, and feeling functions.

Ideally, we use both hemispheres, switching back and forth. It seems that if we could separate the hemispheres, each part would have the special qualities listed in the table below.

Perceptual Qualities of "Left" and "Right" Brain	
"Left Brain"	"Right Brain"
Linear	Spatial
Orderly	Random
Objective	Subjective
Analytical	Intuitive
Mathematical	Artistic
Verbal	Feeling (emotions)
Logical	Sensing
Temporal (time)	Spatial
Detailed	Whole (gestalt)
Physical	Creative
Differentiated	Undifferentiated

From a vision-fitness perspective, I propose that the fovea (looking) triggers a left-brain mode of processing (doing). In a looking mode, or doing state, you have a tendency to be more time-oriented, logical, and verbal. You also tend to be more linear in your thinking, that is, you are focused primarily on one line of thought. From videotaped clinical observations of my patients' faces, I have noted more tension in and around the eye muscles and face while they are looking. You can learn to recognize your own shift to the doing and looking state by noticing times when your breathing becomes shallow, you stare, and your eye muscles, neck, and shoulders become tense.

When you are unable to stay focused (foveal) and tend to be "spacey," you're swinging the balance over to the being state, and you're tending to be more retinal than foveal. This is akin to being more intuitive than analytical. Activities such as art, music, dancing, drawing, and some sports promote a state of being, that is, seeing.

There is a danger when we attempt to tackle activities that promote retinal seeing (accessing the right brain) in a left-brained way. Right-brain activities tend to be fun, light, and often recreational. Being left-brained, that is, analyzing and trying to work it out, can take away the "lightness" of playing a musical instrument, dancing, participating in a sport, painting, or doing photography. The danger, at a physical level, is that the eyes tend to become too foveal when we behave in a left-brained way, and this promotes a drop in natural vision-fitness. The competitive nature promoted by our culture—group sports, making good grades in school, the business world, and keeping up with the neighbors—tends to advance more doing even while participating in being activities. So whatever you are doing, check for shallow breathing, staring, and tension in your eyes. Zoom, and let your eyes dance, and the being state will be reactivated.

Improving your vision-fitness involves teaching your brain and your eyes to maintain an optimum working relationship. Being while doing, and seeing while looking, produces high-level vision-fitness. The vision-fitness lenses mentioned in chapter 3 can assist you in achieving this balance.

Using vision-fitness lenses can help you to alter your control of the brain's hemispheres. I believe that 20/20 lenses tend to generate a more left-brain and doing state. You may notice a desire to talk and explain more when wearing 20/20 lenses. On the other hand, vision-fitness lenses permit you to be with the world; you tend to think less and to observe and see more.

Review the eye anatomy and vision-fitness exercise chart at the end of chapter 4. Breathing, blinking, zooming, crossing your eyes, palming, and using full-spectrum lighting are vision-fitness exercises that can help you to restore a being state while doing.

Chapter 6

Nutrition and Aerobics for Your Eyes

Your vision-fitness can be only as good as the fuel you provide for your eyes and the efficiency of the muscles and organs that circulate blood to them. To achieve maximum vision-fitness, you need to eat foods that enhance your vision and to keep all the body's major muscle groups toned for optimum blood flow and distribution of nutrients.

To simplify complex topics such as nutrition and exercise, I suggest you recall the native African from *The Gods Must Be Crazy*. I am not suggesting that we should return to the life of a Bushman, but we should recognize the value of treating our bodies with the same care and respect as he does. The Bushman metaphor continues to be valid, especially since most of them have excellent vision. Consider his typical day:

Awakening in a primitive hut, he lights a fire and embarks on a one-mile walk to bring enough fresh water to prepare a warm drink for his family. Part of the trip is spent running, and on the return trip, the water is carried on his head or around his neck. Food preparation involves hunting in sunlight, using his eyes and many of his muscles. Food consumption is simple—berries, fruit, a little meat, vegetables, beans, and grains. Time is spent preparing the food and savoring the taste over a lengthy meal with other family members. There's a natural balance of aerobic exercise and small portions of healthy food.

Contrast the Bushman's lifestyle to a typical scenario in your Western lifestyle. You are awakened by an alarm clock—probably when it's still dark. After rolling out of bed, you exercise your finger muscle by switching on the light. Programmed from the night before, the coffee machine has your pick-me-up waiting. You shave (if you do) with an electric razor or you breathe in the chemical fumes of shaving cream as it prepares your stubble for removal. With a flick of a handle, hot water pours from the shower. After dressing, you select a prepared cereal (usually with added sugar and salt), add milk that you bought at a store, and eat a meal, probably while standing. You exercise by walking to your car, train, or bus, in which you travel to your place of work. This modern lifestyle has a bearing on the maintenance and development of your vision-fitness.

While researching the effects of nutrition and exercise on vision-fitness, I subjected myself and other volunteers to many experiments. The results clearly suggest that you can monitor your seeing/looking fitness based on the type of food you eat and the extent of aerobic exercise you perform. During our original research study in 1982, for example, one of the subjects reported a nutrition-related experience that he had during the twenty-one-day experimental period. All the participants eliminated red meat, alcohol, sugar, dairy, and processed foods from their diets. They ate fresh fruits, vegetables, and a minimum of chicken and fish. The use of soy products, beans, and grains was also encouraged.

Eric was following the program diligently. He hadn't worn his strong eyeglasses for eight days; he had given up all coffee and sugar; and his natural vision-fitness level had improved by 30 percent. One night he and his wife went out to dinner, and Eric succumbed to a cup of coffee and a delicious piece of cheesecake. Within thirty minutes Eric's vision-fitness without glasses had dropped so dramatically that his wife had to lead him by the arm from the restaurant.

From the evidence cited in the literature (see the Selected Bibliography) and my communication with researchers around the world, it would appear that the ciliary (focusing) muscles are sensitive to fluctuations in blood-sugar levels. I recall a fourteen-year-old, Pat, who was learning to use natural vision-fitness, thus avoiding strong eyeglasses. Her natural vision-fitness was 76.5 percent. One day Pat arrived at the clinic, where I was conducting vision-fitness training and research, with a soda. Before she was able to drink her soda, I recorded her natural vision-fitness level with both eyes open. I then asked her to drink the soda. Within fifteen minutes, her vision-fitness dropped to 58.5 percent.

Another participant in the research shared this experience:

"For over a week I had restricted my eating to rice, vegetables, a small portion of fish or chicken, fresh fruit, yogurt, and bread. I walk to work each day, and I noticed that through my vision-fitness lenses (83.6 percent), I could see objects, signs, and cars a lot clearer. On the ninth day of the experiment, I stopped at a fast-food place. After consuming scrambled eggs and a roll, I continued the walk to my office. Within twenty minutes, I could hardly see through my reduced-power lenses. I would estimate my vision-fitness dropped to 70 percent. This experience convinced me that what I eat affects my looking."

These kinds of reports are common. The intake of certain foods by sensitive individuals seems to cause an allergic reaction that can be revealed in the functioning of the eyes. It would seem that these sugary and fatty foods trigger a chemical change that is recorded by the eyes.

The foods you eat may affect your vision as a result of the way other organs in your body react to your diet. If your heart, lungs, liver, and kidneys are forced to work overtime processing the food you eat, your eyes will suffer the consequences. For example, the liver purifies the blood before it carries nutrients to the different parts of the body. If you consume fatty foods, the liver has to overwork, and some remaining debris might end up in the blood that ultimately reaches the eyes. In a sense, the blood vessels and other parts in the eyes can be thought of as a dumping ground. The eyes can be only as healthy as the content and purity of the blood.

Exercise, particularly aerobic, causes your heart to pump more blood through the various parts of the body. Consequently, the blood in the eyes is flushed, which stimulates the eyes. The nerves are then better able to send fast and accurate messages.

Over the years, I have received numerous reports from my patients about changes in their vision-fitness percentage while involved in aerobic activity. Long-distance runners report periods of intense clarity without lenses. Students already having natural 100 percent vision-fitness relate how much more they can retain while reading after an aerobic workout. Video-display-terminal operators who exercise at lunchtime experience less eyestrain by the end of the day compared to days when they don't exercise.

A report from a professional tennis player who completed a vision-fitness program further illustrates this point:

"Exercise for me is a form of expanding my rhythm (breath) and the space occupied by my body. As I stretch my body and eye muscles into space, so my ability to see increases. While exercising, I move my eyes left, right, up, and down. I focus to different distances.

"Whenever possible, I wear no lenses while playing; otherwise I slip on my vision-fitness prescription. I have, on a number of occasions, beaten my partner using my natural vision-fitness. It's almost like I can see the moving ball better.

"My warm-up procedure includes swinging my body from left to right, hanging my head down, and rolling my neck. These exercises help me loosen my muscles and keep them flexible. I also monitor my breathing and stretch my eyes. After a vigorous workout, I'll palm my eyes for fifty breaths and visualize the eye parts receiving healthy blood."

We've seen how the Bushman incorporates natural practices of good diet and exercise into his daily schedule. What about your own lifestyle? In the past you've probably been too busy doing to make room for similar practices in your routine. But what we've learned about vision-fitness makes it all the more important that you pay careful attention to the foods you choose to eat and that you set aside time to exercise.

Well Then, What Should I Eat?

This is a complex question. I wish there were a simple formula I could give you. Probably the most effective way for me to make suggestions is to share my personal experiences and experiments. Over the years, I have studied different nutritional approaches to better my own chances for disease prevention and also to increase my vision-fitness. What follows is my personal approach to eating. It is an assimilation of many theories and practical experiences. But first, here are two perspectives that allowed me to be flexible.

A macrobiotic teacher from Japan once said to me:

"If you cannot occasionally drink beer or eat red meat, then your body is sick."

And when questioned about the nutritional principles that contributed to his cancer regression, a cancer patient participating in a natural approach to cancer treatment stated:

"I eat anything my body wants. When I eat an ice-cream sundae, I tell my body to really enjoy the value of this food."

What then, is my philosophy regarding food? I believe in moderation. I prefer a non-fanatical approach to well-being. Preparing even the simplest meal is like creating a work of art. Eating for me is a joy. Food is sacred to me. I feel that if I am in tune with my body, it'll let me know what food it desires. Of course, I have to monitor emotional gratification using nutritionally sound principles.

I do the best I can to avoid producing new belief systems about foods. For instance, a report I read claimed that an overconsumption of dairy products can lead to a change in the metabolism of the lens of the eye, which may later result in a cataract (clouding of the lens).

Based on this report, it would be easy for me to tell you to eliminate dairy products from your diet. Other research states that excessive sugar and simple-carbohydrate intake is bad for the ciliary (focusing) muscle. Do I then suggest giving up sugar and dairy products? I would prefer that you experiment for yourself. I have found that small amounts of dairy products and sugar are OK for me, but you must discover your own tolerance level. Do you know the critical point that will lead to a gradual decrease in your vision-fitness?

With this in mind, here is the dietary approach I use: Grain (rice, millet, quinoa, and buckwheat) and legume (bean) combinations are my staple diet. I also use soybean products such as tofu and tempeh. I add sea vegetables to my grains and soups, and I use miso (soybean paste) at least twice a week as a soup or drink. Free-range chicken and fresh fish, once a week, are supplemented with steamed, pressure-cooked, or stir-fried vegetables, including deep-root varieties such as daikon and carrots. I use small amounts of fresh ginger, garlic, cayenne powder, and other seasoning herbs. I have a fresh salad with live sprouts such as alfalfa.

My liquid intake includes herbal teas, vegetable drinks, and freshly extracted juice from vegetables and, in the summer, from fruit. I eat fruit and drink juice mainly during the summer months. Breads, soy margarine, and homemade preserves are used as special treats.

For breakfast I eat a mixed-grain cereal with soy or rice milk. About once or twice a week, I have scrambled, poached, or soft-boiled eggs and whole-wheat toast. When eating meals out, I'll order an occasional beer and have fresh fish. Sometimes I'll have a dessert.

When I notice a drop in my vision-fitness, I take a multivitamin and mineral supplement that includes extra ascorbate vitamin C, multi B, water-soluble A, and amino-acid chelated zinc.

When you plan your own diet, consider the basics. Remember the four food groups. Cut back a little on dairy products and red meat, and balance the groups.

Using vision-fitness lenses and making use of the biofeedback nature of the eyes, you can monitor which foods affect you. Remember that the effects may be more than just a drop in your vision-fitness percentage. You may experience impaired "two-eyed fitness" (ability of the two eyes to work together). Also, your seeing/

looking balance may be upset. But in time and with patience you'll begin to know what your body requires for maximum general physical fitness and vision-fitness.

| The Nutritional Elements and Their Eye Relationship ||
Eye Anatomy	Nutritional Elements
Sclera (the white of the eyeball)	Calcium
Conjunctiva (the covering of the sclera)	Vitamins B_2, B_{12}, folic acid
Cornea	Vitamin A
Lens	Vitamins C, E, B_2
Ciliary muscle	Chromium
Retina	Vitamin A, zinc, and other minerals
Macula (the area around the fovea)	Vitamin B complex

How Much Should I Exercise?

As a rule of thumb, exercise for fifteen to twenty minutes while your pulse beats between 125 and 145 beats per minute. Again, moderation is the key. A slight perspiration is satisfactory, but don't become so tired that you're panting.

Get in touch with a balance between your being and your doing as you exercise. Your seeing can become more vivid. Your field of vision may widen and colors may become brighter. You may feel as if there is nothing in your way. Your body can feel expansive and open.

Experiment and discover what happens for you with each lifestyle change you make. Nurture your body with good foods and healthy exercise, and your vision will become fit.

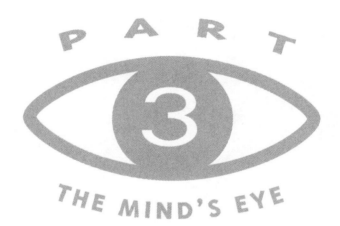

PART

3

THE MIND'S EYE

Chapter 7

Does Your Mind Guide Your Outer Seeing?

Does your state of mind affect your ability to see? To answer this question you might find it helpful to transcend your traditional view of your eyes—that they're bad, that there's a problem, or that you can't see. Attempt to keep an open mind. Begin using the ideas that follow in a self-experiment. In the beginning, your rational mind may wish to dismiss these ideas as impossible. Ask your rational mind to be patient. Be open. Consider Helen Keller's insight:

"The best and most beautiful things in the world cannot be seen or even touched. They must be felt with the heart."

Since the time you stood in line for your eye test at school, you've thought that your eyes are either good or bad. If you "failed" the school eye test, you were told to see an eye doctor. The doctor probably told you that your eyes were weak, long, short, cloudy, or had too much pressure. Blurriness, double vision, eyestrain, cataracts, glaucoma, iritis, nearsightedness, and other eye conditions may have been involved in the diagnosis.

Your mother, father, or other family members probably comforted you by saying that you inherited their "weak" eyes. You solidified the perception that you had a problem. For most of you, each visit to the eye doctor meant further bad news. Your eyes needed a stronger lens prescription, surgery, or medication. The belief that your eyes were bad became further ingrained. Could it be that this thinking contributed to the decreased capability of your eyes to do their job?

Let's think about our aboriginal counterpart again. In the middle of the jungle there are no optometrists or ophthalmologists. If and when the jungle-dweller experiences a problem with his eyes, such as a sore, puffiness, redness, or blurred or impaired vision, he visits the local medicine man or shaman, where, in addition to obtaining a cure, he is encouraged to explore why the gods or spirits are making his eyes the way they are. In a sense, the shaman acts as a teacher by helping the person to determine the cause of the condition. For example, redness with swelling may be metaphorically associated with inner anger or upset. A ritual might follow. Perhaps a natural concoction from vegetation, animal juices, and soil (we would call it a poultice) is given to the person to place on the eye(s). The healing process requires the patient to be an active participant, asking him/her to look at his/her involvement in the eye condition. This approach goes beyond simply treating the symptom or even clearing up the physical condition.

Drawing on this metaphor, you can begin to think of your eye condition as an indication of what is happening in your mind's eye. It's a combination of your thoughts, beliefs, fears, and angers. It also includes perceptions picked up from your parents, siblings, teachers, and others. This is why people don't all develop the same eye conditions. Each of you carries your own unique imprint of past patterns of perception. You visit your traditional eye doctor with a symptom—perhaps blurriness, eyestrain, "floaters," or pain. Your eye doctor examines the eyes and takes various measurements. She then makes a comparison to some norm and informs you whether or not you fit into that norm. If you don't, some remedial measures may be suggested. These are not substantially different from the African ritual, and they usually take the form of eyeglasses, contact lenses, surgery, or medication.

Contrast this familiar approach with that of the modern preventive eye doctor, usually a functional optometrist. Like the shaman, he or she views the physical eye as a mirror of the mind's eye. In effect, your eyes reveal something about your inner perceptions, either past or current. The obvious and ideal situation is to combine Western and traditional shamanistic approaches, use the technology of a vision-fitness lens prescription, and enlist your eye doctor or a suitably trained professional to help you examine the types of perceptions you have in your mind's eye.

A couple of case examples will bring this theory into focus.

Annie, age forty-one, claiming to be bored with life, had detached herself from the world by living in a small cabin in the woods of central Oregon. By isolating herself in the woods, Annie avoided seeing herself in relation to the rest of the world. She had withdrawn from traditional life in order to learn about another part of her being. I was not surprised when she described her physical ailments. Annie had been a diabetic, under control, for many years. (Am I "sweet" enough? Am I liked and accepted as I am?) The foveal area of the retina in both of her eyes had become detached, impairing the retina's function. This resulted in her side vision becoming quite narrow. Behaviorally speaking, Annie had secluded her mind's-eye seeing and detached her willingness to see and clearly participate in life.

I assisted Annie in correlating these observations, and following our first visit she went to have eye surgery. Her new awareness helped Annie to change her vision of her lifestyle. In a way, her mind's eye was retrained to perceive in harmony with the reality seen by the physical eye.

I didn't expect Annie to recover much of her vision-fitness. She did, however, move from a position of despair—one of believing that she was going blind—to a new outlook that enabled her to go back to a small town and successfully continue a home business. Her seeing (vision) improved and her eye condition stabilized.

Obviously, this is an extreme example of the proposition that the mind's eye can influence the physical eye. The point is that if you believe you have an eye "problem," then the "condition" has less chance of "getting better." In Annie's case, after our consultation, she saw her nearsighted eyes and her detachment "condition" as a gift that allowed her to learn something about herself. My intensive case history and video analysis of her previous thinking and destructive inner vision pointed to her mind's-eye perceptions as being one of the causes in her significant drop in vision-fitness. Like the African "patient," Annie took advantage of her situation to gain new insights into how she participated in the development of the eye "gift." She also underwent surgical intervention to prevent her eye condition from getting worse. One could speculate that the surgery alone resulted in her improved perception as well as in her more positive attitude. But I believe the vision-fitness intervention helped her to gain a perspective that facilitated the surgical and natural healing process.

Abe, age thirty-one, had been told by his eye doctor at age sixteen that by the time he was in his mid-thirties, he would need to wear glasses. During his early thirties, Abe made a career change and became a computer programmer. It was at this time that he first noticed blurred vision. His optometrist confirmed Abe's suspicion. His eyes were too long and thus nearsighted. He would need moderately strong eyeglasses. During the next year Abe went through two more changes in prescription, each stronger than the last. By the third pair, Abe consulted me.

During our consultation I asked Abe what else had been happening in his life during the career change. He revealed that eighteen months prior to getting his first pair of glasses, he had ended an eight-year marriage. He reported great fear and anxiety about the future. He couldn't see how he was going to make it financially. His inner vision was one of failure in both his career and his relationships. Abe's intense computer-study programs, his memory of the eye doctor saying he would need glasses in his mid-thirties, and his fear of the future all precipitated the changes in his physical eyes.

My first step was to assist Abe in changing the way he talked about his life. He repeatedly used the word "can't" and the phrase "I don't know." By rephrasing to "I know," he initiated seeing in the future. For example, I would ask Abe questions such as "Where would you like to work?" or "What type of relationship are you looking for?" Since he had internally pro-grammed his mind's eye not to see clearly, he responded to the questions by saying, "I don't know." As long as Abe voiced the words "I don't know," his mind's eye didn't see. After a few sessions, he began to answer these questions by saying, "I would like to work for a high-tech company, and I am interested in a professional woman who loves the outdoors."

These answers helped Abe get clarity in his mind's eye. He asked his friends to remind him whenever he spoke in a negative or unaccountable way. He also used the vision-fitness lenses and incorporated exercises into his daily routine in order to balance his being and doing states.

Soon Abe no longer needed corrective lenses except to drive. He became more outgoing and ended up finding a fabulous job and a mag-nificent relationship—all within a seven-month period.

Each eye condition is representative of a mind's-eye perception. Each condition is a gift, offering a specific lesson. The following guide may help you to discover your particular gift.

Perceptual Understanding of Various Eye Conditions

Eye Condition or "Problem"	Mind's-Eye Perception	Gift or Lesson
Nearsightedness	Fear of seeing the future. Pulling inward to self: "I am afraid to see what's out there."	Reach for your dream. Push outward. Learn about creating space. Confront your power.
Farsightedness	Fear of seeing the present: "I have to see out into the future." Anger toward self or others. Pushing space and people away. Wanting to break out and be independent.	Career or relationship changes may be impor-tant. Learn about commit-ment. Be connected to the present.
Astigmatism	Distortion of one part of your reality. Nearsighted-ness in one particular thread or part of your life. Restriction or fear in one of the ways you see.	Open up to the future in one area of your life. Stretch yourself beyond beliefs of what's possible in a particular part of your seeing.

(continued on next page)

Perceptual Understanding of Various Eye Conditions, cont'd.

Eye Condition or "Problem"	Mind's-Eye Perception	Gift or Lesson
Glaucoma	Feeling filled with internal pressure, as if you're exploding. You're rushed. You're overly inside yourself. You're closed off.	Let go. Be free and flowing.
Macular degeneration	Loss of the central theme of life. Not seeing the point to living: "Spacing out is what life's about."	Reconnect to the central focus of life.
Retinal detachment	Feeling separate, unloved. Losing touch with the outside. Not wishing to see outside your immediate line of vision.	Stay connected with others, particularly outside your immediate sphere of activity.
Cataract	Clouding or blocking out of life. You avoid seeing what there is to look at in your life.	Issues need to be looked at. Clean up the aspects of life that are clouding your view of what's important.
Eye turning	Blocking of energy. Can't-cope mechanism. Life's too much, too complicated for you to deal with.	Learn cooperation and partnership between self and the world. Accept and love self and others.
Inward	Overcompensation or excessive focusing.	Relax and look out.
Outward	Spacing out. Drifting away.	Stay centered. Focus on details.
Lazy eye	Laziness in receiving or expressing vision. Turning off energy. Avoidance of the truth. Unacceptance.	Strive for balance. Open up to your blocks to learning in life.
Corneal conditions	Blocking of power. Fear of loss of power. Seeing pain.	Reclaim personal power and vision.

When you are exercising, driving your car, walking, standing in line, or preparing to go to sleep, see all the parts of your eyes as being healthy. Use "I am" statements to affirm what you wish to see, for example, "As I breathe, I look from my heart, through my eyes, and I see the truth." Dare to dream and to have a vision, whether it be healthy eyes, less eyestrain, less dependency on glasses, a new job, a wonderful vacation, or improved natural vision-fitness. Let your mind's eye orchestrate your physical eye in the direction you choose.

Chapter 8

Events, Experiences, and Decisions: Their Effect on Vision

Let's again imagine that you're an aborigine living in a jungle. Your world consists of a five-mile radius around your home. Since childhood you've been trained in how to survive. You have learned how to move your body skillfully and how to respond to poisonous snakes, hungry lions, and wild game you may wish to capture for food. Your physical eye has a simple view of the world: it consists of the jungle, family members, and your home. Your mind's eye and your thinking are equally uncomplicated. Your inner perceptions of your family and surroundings are peaceful and fearless.

One day while wandering at the edge of the forest, you suddenly arrive at a new place—a view your eyes have never seen before. You see people whose bodies are covered by clothes. They are driving jeeps and carrying guns. Your physical eyes send new information to your mind's eye. These new perceptions are processed in the context of your previous experiences. For example, what is your view of a gun? Since you have no previous experience, your perception is naive. A gun's potential to harm is not in your visual experience. Therefore, you do not fear it. If you then see someone being hurt by a gun, a visual fear response will be activated, and when you see a gun in the future, you'll see it through filters of fear and danger.

I am sure that most of you have not lived in a secluded jungle. But you probably have been exposed to events in your life that have precipitated fear responses. I am suggesting that your mind's eye, out of a survival instinct, has made mental decisions to protect you from some of the things you've seen. Unlike the aborigine, you are exposed to one crisis or stress factor after another, including wars, television, violence, hijackings, restructuring of the family unit, city life, financial challenges, competitive education, alcohol, drugs, AIDS, missing children, threats of nuclear annihilation—and the list goes on. It's not surprising that your physical eye eventually adjusts to these mind's-eye perceptions. There's so much in your world today that you'd rather not see.

Before we can understand how the mind's eye can affect vision, we must first look more closely at the way the mind's eye functions. From the moment you were conceived, even before your eyes were "seeing," your body and brain tissue were storing information about events. For instance, when your mother ate a certain food, your body recorded the event as an experience. If your mother consumed too much sugar, your body experienced certain sensations, and your mind's eye recorded and made a decision about this experience.

After birth, your eyes began to capture these events visually. Your mind's eye is a videotape. Stored in the brain's library is the data of all sensory experiences, that is, everything you've felt, heard, said, and seen. By the time you were six months old, you were more than likely seeing 20/20; by twelve months your two eyes were working together.

Imagine for a moment that you are fourteen months old. Your attention is focused on the bright orange-red color of flames in a fireplace. You maneuver your body over to the fire and begin to play. Very soon you burn your hands and start to cry. You make a decision that red and orange is associated with pain and crying. Your mind's eye records this experience of pain associated with seeing red and orange.

Later you see some brightly colored red and orange paper. Based on your previous experience, you pull away and don't wish to touch the paper. If you continue to respond this way to visually presented red and orange items, the muscles and structures of your eyes learn to see in a fearful way. In effect, your eyes and your vision constrict and become tense. Because of the mind's-eye perception that red and orange burns, it sends fearful messages to the physical eye.

This connection between perception and action is clearly evident when watching eye and facial expressions recorded by a video camera. Certain probe questions stimulate mind's-eye memories of upsetting past events. As you think about those events, tension and fear are reflected in the gestures you make. It's as if your memory of the previous events triggers a survival response. The way you see the present is affected by your records of past information, which is then reflected in the gestures made by your eyes and face.

Consider that the events of your life, along with genetic, physical, nutritional, and environmental factors, may have affected your eyesight. Retrace the events in your life. Is it possible that these events triggered physical and mental perceptions that brought about your present level of vision-fitness? A few telling case studies will illustrate this concept.

For Nancy, age forty-three, the first major life event she could recall was moving from town to a farm at age three. Her mother gave up a career to bring up the family and look after the home. Six months later, Nancy's younger brother was born. An immediate close bond between her brother and mom developed.

During the next two years, Nancy saw her mother become more and more unhappy over giving up her dream to become a concert pianist. During the first grade, Nancy had a routine eye exam and was given a clean bill of health. She continued to observe her mother's unhappiness at being secluded on the farm.

During the year that followed, Nancy began to exhibit "tomboy" behaviors. Her dad even began calling her "Billy." It was in the second grade that she "needed" her first pair of eyeglasses.

Between the ages of eight and fourteen, Nancy deeply resented the close connection between her brother and mother. She and her brother fought constantly. She experienced feelings of abandonment and began to question whether she could trust men.

By age twelve, Nancy's mother expressed the desire to leave Nancy's father. This family change led to much confusion for Nancy, and it created distortions in the way she viewed relationships. During this period her eyeglasses kept becoming stronger. At age twenty-five, Nancy married a man of whom her mother disapproved, and in the following thirteen years, Nancy saw her mother only twice. At age forty-two, her left eye perceived significantly more "blurry" than her right eye.

When I first met Nancy, she was a distressed woman, afraid and withdrawn. During our first few sessions she recognized the correlation of the above experiences and internal decisions with the way her eyes saw her parents' lives: the development of her nearsightedness paralleled the events. She had seen her parents, particularly her mother, as unfulfilled. Nancy found she had replicated that perception in her own life—she lived by herself and felt lonely.

Within a few weeks, Nancy began taking ownership of her life. She set new goals and dreamed new dreams, creating new mind's-eye pictures. She stimulated her physical eyes with fitness exercises and wore vision-fitness lenses. Nancy realized that she could stay stuck in seeing the old way, as a child, or she could make new choices—decisions that would work for her in her adult life.

When Nancy chose to change, her vision-fitness began to improve. At first the fitness gains were fleeting and elusive. Later flashes of clarity lasted for minutes. At times her vision-fitness jumped to 95 percent through her vision-fitness lenses. Other times her fitness dropped to 70 percent when she became stuck in the past. Nancy's eyes are a perfect metaphor of how one's inner vision and outer seeing/looking are connected. Nancy is still on the journey of seeing without glasses, using the vision-fitness lenses and participating in other personal-growth experiences.

Brenda had never needed eyeglasses. When she was nineteen, her brother was diagnosed with cancer and died within six months. Three months after his death, Brenda was diagnosed as nearsighted. Shortly thereafter, her right eye began turning in. Brenda faithfully wore her new glasses, thinking that her eyes would be corrected. Although her ophthalmologist suggested surgery for the turned-in eye, Brenda decided to wait. At age twenty-one, Brenda took a new job that proved to be very stressful. After eight hours of desk work, her right eye was tired and turned in even more.

Two years later, Brenda heard about the research I was conducting and asked to participate. She expressed concern that her friends at work were teasing her about her "funny" eye. The first step was to get her into vision-fitness contact lenses. (Brenda wouldn't wear eyeglasses.) After two months of vision-fitness exercises, Brenda started to see out of both eyes for short periods of time. One day, while engaged in strenuous physical exercise, Brenda screamed out her frustration. She happened to look up at an eye chart and screamed again. Her vision-fitness had increased 40 percent. She then consulted a social worker with whom I was collaborating in the research. Brenda learned that she had blocked her self-expression after her brother died. She had become introverted and difficult to be with. Six more months passed, and Brenda was making steady progress. She showed more signs of using both eyes together, her self-image was improving, and she was becoming more successful in her job. However, the pressure at her job also increased. It became unbearably difficult for her to handle the teasing when her eye did turn in. Brenda left the vision-fitness program.

One year later, I met Brenda again. She had undergone surgery to have her right eye "straightened." Because she had had the vision-fitness training, both of her eyes were working together. As we parted, she expressed herself loudly: ". . . and I'm getting married next month!"

Like Nancy and Brenda, your present level of vision-fitness may be influenced by events in your past that triggered fearful or limiting eye and mind perceptions. However, you can remove any "filters" you may have placed over your inner vision. As an exercise, find a quiet place where you can close your eyes. While breathing and relaxing your body parts, go back in time through the videotape library of events in your mind's eye. (An alternative exercise is to do the procedure before sleeping. Let your dreams tell you about pertinent events.) Look for events that are positive and negative. Identify experiences that may have precipitated fear responses and decisions made by your mind's eye to protect you. A good rule of thumb is to look back twelve to eighteen months prior to having eye symptoms or getting eyeglasses. When you open your eyes, explore the signifi-cance of what you've seen. How do your previous mind's-eye pictures relate to your present level of vision-fitness?

Now you're ready to generate new events. Plan to have some exciting new experiences that will stimulate you to make new deci-sions about what you currently see. Make a list of recreational, work, home, family, and relationship "things" you'd like to do. Choose events that provide feelings of completion, that are fun, and that are different. Challenge yourself by not wearing your eyeglasses or con-tacts. If your vision-fitness is low, wear vision-fitness lenses. You might call your parents and tell them that you love them, contact an old friend, see a good movie, go skiing, take sailing lessons, plan a vaca-tion, browse through a bookstore, or go dancing.

See if you can experience every new event in your life as a gift. Find out what there is to learn in everything you see. Monitor your vision-fitness during each new experience. Remember to love your "blur."

Chapter 9

Fear and Anger: Their Effect on Vision

We've seen that the events and experiences you've had and the resulting decisions you've made are factors that can keep you from seeing as well as you otherwise would (see chapter 8). I believe fear and suppressed anger are the common denominators responsible for the impact of these events. These emotions are thought to be stored both mentally and physically. It had been difficult for me to comprehend how experiencing fear and/or anger alters one's vision-fitness until optometrist Robert Pepper introduced me to the idea of working with patients on a large trampoline.

Let's imagine you are having a session with me. You are wearing comfortable clothes, and you remove your eyeglasses or contacts. You see a large trampoline in the center of a large room with a vaulted ceiling. You climb up on the trampoline and begin to jump up and down, moving your arms in small circles in front of you. After a reminder, you become aware of your shallow breathing. You notice that your eyes are riveted to one place. Your eye, neck, and shoulder muscles feel tight. You might also notice if the new situation produces fearful and tight feelings in your chest and stomach.

After a short while you begin to master the trampoline bounce and you relax. You look around and notice an increase in your natural vision-fitness. As you smile, you hear the next instruction: "Now do a seat drop and then a knee drop." Again, your initial body reaction is to tighten. As you imagine doing a seat drop, you sense a fear of falling. You might think to yourself: "You're crazy; I can't do that." I invite you to observe your defensiveness and anger.

Our imaginary exercise continues, and the fear/anger pattern is repeated with each new instruction:

- "Count from one to ten on every bounce, and do a knee drop on two and a seat drop on eight."

- "Same as before, but now clap your hands on five and say 'Relax.'"

- "Now count backward from ten to one, and let two become eight, eight become five, and five become two."

Did our imaginary trampoline session produce any actual sensations of fear or anger within your body? If so, you have experienced how overload in your mind's eye produces fear. It's the fear of the unknown, the fear of failure and rejection. In most of your life situations, thoughts and feelings of fear and the resulting muscular tensions go unnoticed, but those feelings, even if they are not acknowledged, ultimately reach the muscles of your eyes. These muscles can become tense and can spasm.

A real trampoline experience is one way to help yourself become aware of the way in which your thoughts and feelings affect your body and especially your eyes. Then you can train your eyes using the vision-fitness program outlined in chapter 12. Your vision-fitness percentage will increase as you master the program. If you were actually to bounce up and down performing mind's-eye exercises and monitoring all the variables (on two do a knee drop, call out a number on every other bounce, on five clap your hands, on eight do a seat drop, and remember to breathe and blink), you'd find that there's not enough time to think about anything but the present. Being present in the here and now is the important variable. If you start thinking about the past or worrying about the future, your present "being" state breaks down. When this happens, your performance also breaks down. So your breakdown in performance serves as feedback, a reminder whenever you leave the present. Your response to these "breakdowns" lets you experience your inner fears or suppressed anger.

After four hours of work on a trampoline, farsighted Jill, age sixteen, reported the following:

"I'm amazed at how frustrated I become when I can't do something as simple as jumping up and down and spelling a word. When you reminded me to breathe and feel what was going on inside of me, I suddenly screamed out, just like I want to do at my mother. After the session, I felt relieved. My body and eyes were relaxed. I could center my eyes closer to my nose and read more comfortably."

My clinical observations and personal experience of this phenomenon suggest that if you are nearsighted you probably spend a lot of time examining the past in your mind's eye, looking at those old events, experiences, and decisions. You have developed a repertoire of reasons explaining why you are the way you are and why you see the way you do. It's as if your physical eye is trying to see at your current age, but your mind's eye is still living in the fear and anger of the past. Alternatively, if you are farsighted you probably spend a lot of time worrying about how you'll do in the future.

How then can you see now? You must learn to stay in the present while also being aware of where you've been and where you are going. When you relax your mind's-eye thinking and your body and eye muscles, you are more in the present. Bringing your mind's eye into the present can help you to increase your vision-fitness percentage, develop greater use of the two eyes, and enhance your memory and reading ability.

Another way to accomplish this is through what Robert Pepper calls "visual mapping." In visual mapping you develop a mental plan, a strategy of what to do. Once this map is established in your mind's eye, your physical seeing can be orchestrated in a relaxed way. Take the word *Louisiana*. Imagine jumping on the trampoline while spelling this word without any visual map or rehearsal. If you have to think about how to spell *Louisiana*, you'll use too much energy thinking. Your attention will be taken away from "being" with jumping and seeing. Then you will fail to monitor your physical-eye looking in a relaxed way.

You can avoid this disrupting distraction by working out a visual map ahead of time. You might consider breaking up the word into three segments: (1) LOU, (2) ISI, and (3) ANA. With your eyes closed, imagine seeing frame 1, LOU, and then frames 2 and 3. When your mind's-eye picture is clear, imagine jumping on the trampoline again. Now imagine frame 2, then 1, and finally 3. How flexible are you in manipulating three frames in your mind's eye? Notice if you're straining to see. By using visual mapping when you jump and spell at the same time, you won't throw yourself out of balance in an effort to do two things at once.

You can use the same approach with objects in your world, either without eyeglasses or while wearing your vision-fitness lenses. The Eye-C charts (see chapter 12) can also be used the same way. Allow your mind's eye to see clearly via visual mapping. For example, picture your favorite store where you purchase fruits and vegetables. Imagine that your refrigerator is empty and you're walking down the store aisles selecting juicy apples, red tomatoes, green celery, and orange carrots. See the rows of priced produce. Or, while driving down the freeway, see the sign for your exit clearly in your mind's eye. What is the color, shape, distance, and size of the sign? Repeat the activity using the Eye-C charts. Without straining, see the edges of the letters, look at the white spaces, and recall the letters from your memory. Use visual mapping to extend your visual imagination. In that way you will develop confidence in your present seeing. You will keep fear and anger responses from creeping into your present. In turn, you'll stay more in the present.

Discussing the way in which fear and anger are related to vision-fitness brings to mind some fascinating research on multiple personalities. Researchers have found that people with split personalities need different eyeglass prescriptions for each of their respective personalities, which means that the person's vision-fitness is different for each personality state.

With this in mind, you might consider the vision-fitness lenses as a way to put yourself in a different "personality state." The slight blur can in some cases frustrate you or even bring up buried fear or anger. Sometimes you may feel as if you're not yourself, as if you are another person. My patients report that this way of seeing allows them to access past events and experiences in the brain (the mind's eye), especially traumatic or fear-based events. For example:

When George was twelve years old, he witnessed his brother's death in a car accident. The incident terrorized him. Approximately twelve months after the accident, George's eyes were measured as nearsighted. At age twenty-five, George began a vision-fitness program.

The physical vision-fitness exercises produced relaxation of the eye muscles. After several sessions, George noticed that following physical labor and release of tension, he had flashes of clear seeing.

At this time George's fear of accidents and his anger toward the driver who caused his brother's death surfaced. He worked through the old feelings. Today, George can legally drive without corrective lenses and has since learned to appreciate the gifts that resulted from his brother's death.

The release of suppressed fear and anger can, indeed, allow you to experience greater vision-fitness. For this stage of the vision-fitness program, it is very important to have a trained person assist you. Counselors, psychologists, psychiatrists, psychotherapists, vision therapists, Bates teachers, vision educators, and rebirthers are good resources. Ask a friend to be a support person as well. Keep a diary of the feelings, thoughts, dreams, or breakthroughs you have. This will be your record of your progress.

In *Love Is Letting Go of Fear*, Gerald Jampolsky wrote, "Seeing is looking with love."

Chapter 10

Right Eye, Left Eye

More than likely you and your eye doctor assume that your eyes will work in harmony if there is a clear image on each fovea. In my experience, this is accurate only if you're like the aborigine we've been discussing, who uses his eyes in myriad ways as he moves through the jungle. The moment you tend toward left-brained, central-foveal looking, undue stress is created in the coordination of the two eyes. You don't use your eyes as an aborigine does, so as you explore these vision-fitness principles, you'll probably notice that each of your eyes has a particular kind of vision.

In Chinese medicine, the right side of the body is associated with expression (left-brain control). The left side is more receiving (right-brain control). If you take this concept a step further, your right eye (which I think of as a channel) extends you, and therefore your vision, out into the world. Your left eye receives visual information from the world. As partial evidence, consider that we know that the sides of the face, as well as the eyes, do not precisely match each other. Studying eyes and faces on video has aided me in guiding my patients to better understand the dynamics of the right-eye/left-eye relationship.

As an exercise, take out your contacts or remove your eyeglasses. Look out of a window at a faraway object, even if it's blurry. Keeping both eyes open, cover one eye and then the other. Repeat until you can sense whether you perceive more out of one channel than the other. Begin thinking of your eyes as a channel for energy, as if there's a laser beam traveling outward from the right eye and inward through the left eye. Notice whether you think one eye is good or bad; begin eliminating such judgments. Refer to your "stronger eye" as the greater perceiving channel and the other as the channel that's learning to perceive greatly. This shift in thinking will assist your mind's eye.

By now you have a sense that your perceptions are either different or equal between your two eyes. If there's a difference, you can begin exploring possible reasons why you perceive less clearly in one channel.

Some additional principles of Eastern medicine may be helpful. If the left channel is connected to the right brain, then, according to Chinese philosophy, it is possible that the left eye is the feminine eye. Following this line of thinking, the way you use your left eye reflects the way you see your creativity, your feelings, your ability to receive love and to visualize, and your broad view of femininity. The opposite would be true of the right eye. The way you perceive through your right eye is indicative of the way you see your self-expression, logic, analytical skills, intellectual ability, and verbal skills.

If this is true, the ramifications are phenomenal. What would happen if you covered your greater perceiving channel for a few hours per day? Would you suddenly access the emotions mentioned in chapter 9? Could your seeing and looking improve? If your vision-fitness did improve, would the brain qualities associated with that eye also change? Or is it the other way around—would development of the qualities associated with one side of the brain produce an increase in vision-fitness in the corresponding eye? It might be that in order to improve your vision-fitness at the level of the physical eye, you would first need to make a shift in the type of thinking associated with that eye.

Beth, age thirty-two, was a successful lawyer. When she was a law school student in her late twenties, Beth noticed that the vision in her left eye was blurry. Six years earlier she had been prescribed glasses, but she used them only for movies and night driving. She consulted her eye doctor and was told that her left eye had developed an astigmatism (unequal curvature on the cornea). Full-time use of eyeglasses was prescribed.

By the time Beth consulted me several years later, the astigmatism had worsened. Recognizing that astigmatism is a form of distortion, I helped Beth to look at her distortions concerning her femininity. During law school, she had been one of only three women in a class of forty. Beth felt that she had been groomed to assume a masculine role as a lawyer. She arrived at the realization that she'd never had a real example of how to be an assertive woman. For lack of a better role model, she had patterned herself after her male classmates.

Beth's vision-fitness sessions made use of a patch over her right eye. She explored receiving through her left channel and expressing herself and her female qualities. Over time her vision-fitness percentage improved to a level equivalent to that of age twenty-nine. As Beth developed her vision-fitness, she no longer needed to wear her glasses full time. Her relationship improved and she reported feeling more balanced.

Let's take this idea of gender roles and visual orientation a little further. The model of masculinity in this culture is that of the aggressive, left-brained, intellectual, clear communicator. If you blocked or didn't accept your primary male role model—namely, your father—then it is possible that your right eye might reflect this as a drop in vision-fitness. The left eye would then reflect the opposite—your mind's-eye perceptions of your mother and your feminine viewpoint. The degree to which your two eyes work together, as measured by vision-fitness, might reflect the balance of masculine and feminine attributes in your personality.

Angela was five years old when she and her mother first visited me. Her father had left them when Angela was two. At age three, she developed a turning-in of the right eye. The medical diagnosis was lazy eye complicated by farsightedness. Once glasses were prescribed, the eyes looked cosmetically straight. But after a few weeks, Angela's right eye would turn in even more when her eyeglasses were removed. This continued for the next year. Angela's mother was concerned that her daughter's natural vision-fitness seemed to be decreasing the more she relied on eyeglasses.

My findings confirmed her suspicion. In order to break the dependency, I ordered a vision-fitness lens prescription of one-third less lens power for Angela. Using advanced vision-fitness exercises (see chapter 12), Angela learned how to continually activate the foveas of both eyes.

During the next two years, Angela and her mother consulted me periodically. During that time we uncovered deep feelings of resentment toward her father for leaving. Also, she had few male role models who could have helped her learn how to express her own masculine side. Thus, she learned to suppress this maleness. Her quiet, timid, and fearful behavior reflected this imbalance.

Armed with this awareness, her mother, teachers, and friends supported Angela in developing this part of her personality. She also continued to practice vision-fitness exercises. By the time Angela reached her seventh birthday, she was able to use both eyes at all distances without lenses. Her right eye hardly ever turned in. She was doing well in school and was increasingly expressive. Her mother reported that Angela was much more balanced.

To create greater balance in your own vision, consider speaking with your eye doctor about wearing a patch over your greater perceiving channel. (First, read the section on patches in chapter 12.) You could also tape a makeshift patch over the vision-fitness lens corresponding to that eye. My research suggests that it is best to wear the patch for four hours continuously. You may want to build up to the optimum time in increments of thirty minutes. Of course, you should wear the patch only during non-life-threatening situations. Start off inside, doing dishes, reading, and so on. Later, venture outside. Many of my patients have attempted to play catch and other sports with their greater perceiving channel covered. If your vision-fitness percentage is 100 percent, you can still wear a patch to emphasize the part of the brain you wish to stimulate.

Some of my patients have incorporated the vision-fitness patch idea into their careers:

Sylvia, age forty-four, is a pianist. Her natural vision-fitness is 100 percent, but she tends to use her right eye more than her left. When playing the piano, Sylvia also favors her right hand. Her left hand tends to push too lightly on the keyboard.

After using a patch on her right eye for four hours a day during twenty-one days consecutively, Sylvia's playing changed significantly. When she was more able to balance her looking between both eyes, the balance carried over to her fingers and hands. Sylvia still uses the patch whenever she feels an imbalance.

When you remove the patch, do it slowly. Light will seem quite bright. Notice the colors. Feel how great it is to have both eyes open again. Do you now fully appreciate the value of having two eyes? You'll probably feel a lot more balanced. This increased vision-fitness will show up in your ability to be more effective using your eyes in work, reading, and sports. Recheck to determine whether or not the difference in perception between your two eyes has lessened. How do you feel? Record any physical or emotional responses while wearing the patch. Share your results with someone.

Remember: Your two eyes are wonderful!

Chapter 11
Whole-Brain Processing

Whole-brain processing is your ultimate control of your mind's-eye seeing and physical looking. It's a relaxing unification of the right-eye/left-eye channels. Whole-brain processing is a way to fully accept yourself. It helps you to see your past as the preparation for where you are now and to realize that what you see now is a reflection of your past. Tomorrow's vision can be anything you desire. Acknowledge your perfection and let your eyes see.

In earlier chapters you had the opportunity to relearn how to use each eye separately. You've also monitored your vision-fitness in each eye. The next step is to let your brain learn how to comfortably unite the two channels. This is the highest level of vision-fitness. It's the acceptance of all the forces at work within you. Like the other exercises, whole-brain processing can be performed both at the level of your physical eye and at the mental level of your mind's eye.

The vision-fitness exercises in this chapter will teach you to feel and see what it's like when both eyes work together as a team. Remember to practice the routines with minimal effort and strain, and continue breathing, blinking, and stretching the eye muscles. In other words, don't "try" to do the exercises. Let the exercises guide you to experience the feeling of your eyes working as a team. Do changes in your thoughts, posture, the time of day, and lenses allow you to perceive differently? Use the vision-fitness exercises to get to know yourself and your visual style. There's no right or wrong way to do the exercises. They are simply a means for you to find out what it's like to be in a whole-brain mode of processing.

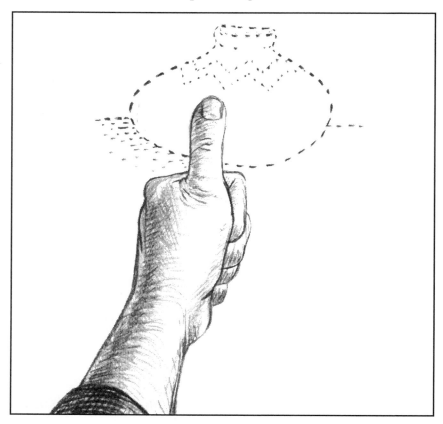

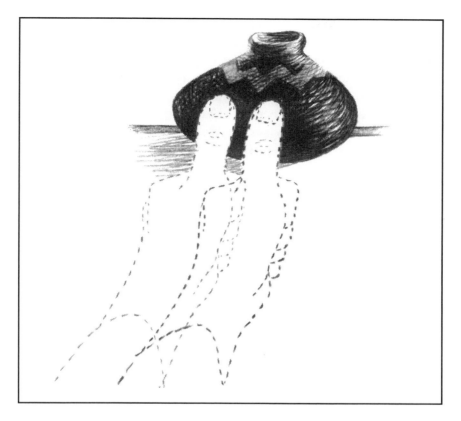

Thumb Zapping Game

Seat yourself comfortably in a chair with your back supported. You may either wear your lenses or go without. Position your hand with your thumb extended in front of your eyes, slightly below your line of seeing. Look at your thumb. Are you aware of your breath? Are you staring at your thumb? Blink and breathe, and while still looking at the thumb, notice everything around the thumb. Your eyes will be focusing on the thumb and turning in (centering). Your thumb will appear in relatively sharp focus (foveal looking) while the background will be blurred (retinal seeing).

Now focus on an object farther away. Notice whether the thumb now has a double image, that is, two thumbs. If not, blink and cover one eye, then the other, until two thumbs appear. (If you have a "lazy" eye, you may not notice two thumbs. Your brain might have learned to shut off the image from one of the eyes.) Observe whether each thumb image is clear. When you can see two distinct thumbs, it is an indication of whole-brain processing at work. Are the thumbs different sizes? Experiment by zooming your focus to a distant object and back. If you alter your focusing distance can you get the thumbs to be the same size? What happens when you wear a patch over the eye that perceives the clearer thumb? When you look at the thumb with both eyes open again, are they different sizes? What is the effect of breathing, standing, standing on one foot, and lying down on the way you see the thumbs? Notice whether one thumb is higher than the other. What happens if you move your left ear toward your left shoulder? Does the higher thumb now look higher or lower? The posture of your head will affect how well the input from each eye is accepted by the brain. If you read in bed or lie on your side, your two-eyed vision-fitness will decrease, and your whole-brain processing will be less effective.

Once you've mastered maintaining an image of two relatively clear thumbs, pick up a book. Place your thumb halfway between the page and your eyes. While reading the printed page, move your thumb wherever your eyes go. Notice that when both eyes are being used (and two thumb images are perceived), you can see all the words on the page. Experiment by closing one eye. Observe that some of the words disappear because the remaining thumb blocks out part of your seeing. Let the thumb corresponding to the lesser perceiving channel lie over the words you're reading. Remember, if both eyes are working together, you will perceive two thumbs. If one of those thumbs goes away, blink, breathe, and look far away, then observe whether the disappearing thumb returns. Keep blinking, breathing, and palming your eyes.

If you get into too much of a "doing" state, you might notice that one of the thumbs disappears, and the remaining thumb may cover the word(s) you're attempting to read. This indicates a shift toward just left- or right-brain processing. This stressful imbalance results when the input from one of the eye channels is not being accepted by the brain.

Periodically during your day, let the thumb-zapping vision-fitness exercise verify your level of whole-brain seeing. Breathe, blink, and palm your eyes in order to remain whole-brained.

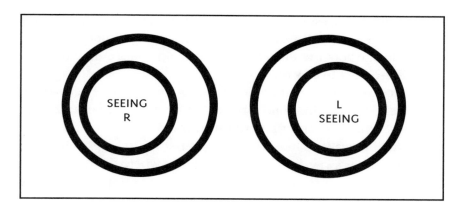

Circles Game

Recall what it feels like to cross your eyes. Position this book so that the circles in the illustration are about sixteen inches in front of your eyes. Cross your eyes ever so slightly until there appear to be three circles. They may be quite blurry. Breathe regularly, and cross your eyes a little more or less. Does the blurriness increase or decrease? Repeat this process. Zoom your eyes between a faraway object and the illustration until the middle picture appears clear. What do you see?

Depending on your level of vision-fitness, you may see the middle picture in one of the following ways:

- An outer and inner circle

- The word SEEING

- The word SEEING, but some of the letters disappear or run into each other

- The word SEEING with an L on the top and an R on the bottom in line with each other

- The L and the R move off center, swimming back and forth

- The inner circle appears to float toward you

As your vision-fitness fluctuates, the way you perceive will also change. An optimum two-eyed (whole-brain processing) level of vision-fitness will result in a perfectly clear inner picture. You'll see a stable L and R and the word SEEING. The letters will not move. You will be able to zoom to different distances and then re-aim your eyes and still see the three pictures.

Once you've mastered the eye-crossing phase, you'll be ready to do the exercise in the opposite way. This time look far away and introduce the target from a position below your line of vision. You might tend to want to look at the target, but try to keep your attention focused far away. You'll discover a point where the three circles will appear. Answer the questions as before and explore the different phases of vision-fitness and perception you experience.

This vision-fitness exercise will teach your eye-crossing (centering) muscles to work in partnership with your eye-focusing (ciliary) muscle. Usually when the eye-crossing muscles lack vision-fitness, you'll automatically overfocus, which can trigger development of nearsightedness or astigmatism.

How flexible is your vision-fitness? Can you form an image of three circles by crossing your eyes and then looking far away? Alternate back and forth. Remember to incorporate breathing, blinking, yawning, and stretching your eye muscles. After five or ten minutes of practicing, palm your eyes.

Mind's Eye Game

The next best thing to a trampoline is a rebounder or minitrampoline. If you have access to one of these bouncers, practice the exercises described in chapter 9 while jumping. You will develop your mind's-eye seeing. Do not do seat and knee drops, of course, since the mat is too small!

Arrows Game

Duplicate the arrows illustration on the next page and place it on a wall. Stand or sit, without corrective lenses, at a distance where you can just make out the directions of the arrows. You'll be at what I call the "blur zone." For some of you this may be ten inches or closer, while for others it may be ten or twenty feet. Place equal weight on both feet if you're standing. Take three deep breaths.

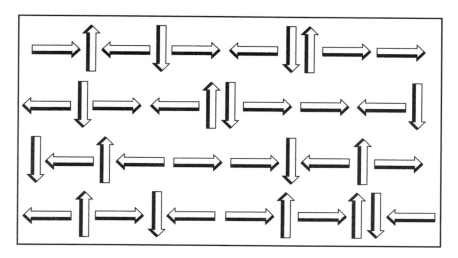

Step 1 Begin at the top left corner and call out the direction of each arrow. Do you move your arms? Do you move your head? Is your rhythm smooth? Are you aware of your breathing? Do you strain to see the arrows? Do your head and neck stretch forward? (*NOTE: Continue to answer these questions for each of the following steps.*)

Step 2 Now call out and use your arm to point in the direction you are saying. Now do it backward from right to left.

Step 3 Use your right hand for pointing to the right, left hand for left, right hand for up, and left hand for down.

Step 4 Do the reverse of Step 3.

Step 5 In your mind's eye, imagine that the arrow has rotated a quarter turn counterclockwise. Say that direction without pointing your arms and hands. Observe whether there are any changes in your rhythm. Later, have a friend or family member clap his/her hands in rhythm; each time you hear the clap, call out the rotated direction. Observe how the clapping paces you. Do you maintain the same level of whole-brain processing, or does a breakdown occur?

Step 6   Repeat Step 5, but now point your hands as you say the direction.

Step 7   Repeat Step 5, but now point your hands in the direction that you see the arrow pointing. Record what feelings are present in your body. How do you respond? Do you get flustered, give up, or simply view the exercises as a challenge?

The arrows exercise is particularly helpful for people who have been told that they have learning disabilities or are dyslexic. The whole-brained nature of the exercise will teach you how to handle overload. Mastery of each step probably stimulates more nerve connections in the brain. It's not uncommon for my patients to report having a headache after the arrows exercise. I recall a teenager saying that it felt like the right side of her head was on fire after this exercise. (If you experience a similar sensation, palm your eyes and discontinue the exercise.)

The more you let go, or just "be," the higher your level of whole-brain processing. Give up analyzing for a while. Trust your mind's eye and intuition. Let the exercise flow. Vision-fitness exercises can be practiced whenever you have the desire to escape your daily routine. Stay with the exercises for at least five minutes but no longer than one hour. The results will include improved efficiency, greater clarity in communication, less eyestrain, improved athletic ability, and less dependency on eyeglasses. Where in your daily life can you use these feelings of "whole-brainedness"?

Enjoy your new vision!

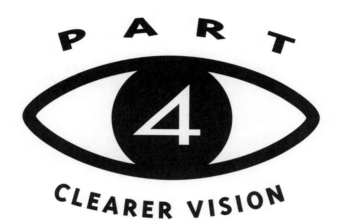

PART

4

CLEARER VISION

Chapter 12

Improving Your Eyesight in Three Phases

The three-phase vision-improvement program that follows was researched as a clinical study. (See the Appendix for a summary of the research.) Its components are designed to work together synergistically when the entire program is practiced as outlined in this chapter. However, let your individual needs and situation determine your level of involvement. You may wish to select or adapt specific exercises to meet a particular vision challenge. If so, I recommend that you flip back to the beginning of the book and reread the material titled "How to Use This Book." Then read chapter 12 once through in order to familiarize yourself with all your options. The listing of "Vision Games for Specific Vision Challenges" (see page 100) may be especially helpful.

The three-phase total-involvement program calls for a high degree of commitment. At first, when you see how much there is to "do" each day, you might feel overwhelmed. Remember, however, that the purpose of the activities is to produce new, relaxed vision habits. There is an inherent risk that you will "try" and "do" the program in an intense way—and fall into the "no pain, no gain" trap. *Seeing Without Glasses* is indeed based on a fitness model, but aerobic and other fitness researchers are finding that brief non-strenuous activities are healthier than prolonged stress-inducing ones. Likewise, your eyes and mind's eye will benefit from a relaxed involvement in the games, which will allow you to use your eye muscles and vision in a more natural and balanced way.

Rather than thinking of the activities as eye exercises, imagine that they are games. In this way you will stimulate the fun of right-brain activity, which in turn will enhance whole-brain functioning.

The rationale for the three-phase program is that it takes approximately twenty-one to sixty days to imprint a new behavior or to break an old habit. Your brain is accustomed to one way of seeing the world. Now you must re-educate your brain in an orderly way that will enable new patterns of seeing to emerge.

Choose activities and vision games that you can practice for fifteen minutes every day. The process is developmentally sequenced. Each new level will increase your visual awareness and participation. Each of the three phases will mark a transition to a more balanced mode of seeing.

One of the most important findings of my research studies was that patients really benefit from support during the program. Find someone who can support you. Ask this person to share your highs and lows, to listen and encourage you when you are down and to celebrate the up times. Your support person can be a counselor, eye doctor, friend, spouse, or therapist.

Again, doing more or trying harder is not necessarily better. Be awake, consistent, and aware. Choose a period when you will have time and be relaxed enough to implement the program.

Choose your degree of participation, remembering that vision-fitness develops when there is a balance between being and doing. Focus on the activities that will promote relaxation, balance, and flow in your life. If you catch yourself worrying about things you haven't done, take a deep breath and modify your goals and the program. Seeing without glasses occurs with minimal effort. Have fun, laugh, and play!

The Three-Phase Activities

Before you undertake the three-phase adventure, familiarize yourself with all of its components. The purpose of the program is to retrain vision-fitness on as many levels as possible. For example:

- Setting goals will bring forth your "dream," first into a vision and then into tangible "sight."

- Using affirmations that address your vision and personal goals will bring your thinking and mind's-eye perceptions into alignment with your desired results.

- Listening to a relaxation tape will alter and balance your brain-wave patterns in order for you to use "whole-brain" perception. You can reprogram your thought patterns in the deepest cells of the brain.

- Eating better-balanced foods will alter the quality of the nutrients arriving at your eyes. The structures of the eye will receive therapeutic levels of vitamins and minerals.

- Exercise will reduce tension in the muscles and improve blood flow.

- Spending time in natural light without eyeglasses or contacts will activate the part of the brain associated with natural light assimilation.

- Wearing the one-eyed patch will modify your perception through one of your eyes. Wearing the two-eyed patch will create greater awareness of peripheral vision and enhanced clarity of sight without corrective lenses.

- Practicing eye-fitness games will increase your awareness of the eye structures, reduce tension and strain, and improve visual and overall body functioning.

- Recording your daily responses will give you feedback on your progress.

Following is a more in-depth description of the program elements. Get a sense of what each part of the plan entails before you actually begin the program. Some of the activities might be easy because you are aware of the process, while others might be more challenging. Be realistic when you set your goals. It is usually wiser to slowly build up your involvement in each activity.

Setting Goals and Defining
What You Wish to See

When I think of goals I am reminded of the distinction between a purpose and a goal. Your purpose is long-term, such as taking a trip to China. The goals that you would need to accomplish in order to make this trip would be to plan the finances, purchase the tickets, decide what to take, and read about the culture.

I view vision-fitness in the same way. First, dream or have a vision about your ultimate purpose. Maybe it is giving up eyeglasses altogether or retaking your driver's test and passing without needing eyeglasses.

You may wish to improve your natural eyesight and still use weaker eyeglasses. Some of you might envision finding a new career, reducing eyestrain, protecting your children's vision, or developing your physical fitness.

Each of these purposes has shorter measurable returns. I like to get the short-term goals in sight and see some outcome. Picture your purpose as being associated with peripheral seeing (which has to do with the retina and a future "vision"), and your goals—immediate specific results—with your looking (which has to do with the fovea and what you can begin to see now). Recall that foveal eyesight (looking) allows you to identify present aspects of your life. The retina (vision) permits observation of future or more peripheral aspects of your seeing. Everything you want to accomplish in life begins with defining a purpose and setting goals. Here is your chance to begin that process for your vision and dreams (purpose) and for the more immediate goals of life.

At the beginning of the three-phase process, write down your long-term purpose and short-term goals for career, work, relationships, money, eyes, vision, diet, and exercise. The career/work distinction is to assist those of you who may wish to make career changes. Relationships and money are included since many of my patients have made positive strides in these directions while they were improving their eyesight. For example, one of your long-term purposes might be to secure a job in a helping profession, which would be supported by the short-term goal of investigating a master's program. Following is a chart that will help you outline your purposes and goals.

Your Purposes and Goals

Career

_____

_____

_____

_____

_____

_____

_____

Work

_____

_____

_____

_____

_____

_____

_____

Relationships

_____

_____

_____

_____

_____

_____

_____

Money

_____

_____

_____

_____

_____

_____

_____

Eyes

_____
_____
_____
_____
_____
_____
_____

Vision

_____
_____
_____
_____
_____
_____
_____

Diet

_____
_____
_____
_____
_____
_____
_____

Exercise

_____
_____
_____
_____
_____
_____
_____

Affirmations

One way to modify your thinking and the way your mind's eye perceives is to use affirmations. Affirmations are positive statements that are usually written or stated aloud. At first you might find the exercise silly or doubt its value. The goal is to repeat an affirmation until there is an inner shift from negative thinking to positive.

Think of an affirmation as adding new software to your brain. In response to the affirmation, your conscious mind might first say: "No!" or "It's blurry—I can't see!" Yet the new software will be recorded on the "silicon chip" of the unconscious. The new data will eventually register at the conscious level.

For example: A patient with 20/80 eyesight, or 58.5 percent vision-fitness, may affirm: "I will pass my driver's test in one month." The patient's first inner response might be: "No way!" After a few times the response might be: "Well, it's possible." Later still the feeling might become: "Yes! I am going for it." The brain/mind's-eye relationship has shifted. Now the possibility exists for the patient to reach her goal.

Stand in front of the Eye-C chart (see page 108) while saying your affirmations. Record the visual responses to the affirmations as + (improved sight), neutral (no change), and – (decreased sight). The affirmations that have a positive effect on your seeing are already coded positively in the brain cells. These affirmations can be used to further enhance your vision when you experience the natural blur, or the blur through your vision-fitness lenses, becoming more intense. Don't give up on the affirmations that produce neutral or negative results. Perhaps your unconscious is resisting the intended message of these affirmations. Incorporating them into the three-phase program will modify your unconscious perception of the affirmation into a positive feeling.

Following are some affirmations that you can use for this program. Whether you choose from among these or make up your own, use affirmations that address your vision and goals. State the affirmation frequently throughout the day, especially while you play the vision games, wear patches, exercise, or prepare meals.

My vision is improving every day.

I am reducing my dependency on eyeglasses in every way.

My sight is improving.

I am in touch with why I block my perception.

I enjoy the way I see.

I love my blur.

I am embracing my blur each day.

I am having fun exploring my blur.

I look forward to seeing less blur.

I am enjoying the way I look and see.

Vision is my creating the way I see.

I now see the truth.

I see the beauty of life.

I forgive my parents' perceptions.

I see the truth of my early environment.

When I see the truth of my upbringing, I feel free.

It is OK for my eyes to see.

I am focusing my perception on my visions.

I am conscious of how my state of being aids my vision.

I am in touch with what I see in my blur.

I like the softness in the way I see.

My mind's eye guides my outer sight.

I am powerful, and I am healing my eyes.

I feel less vulnerable without my eyeglasses.

I have clear and healthy vision.

I am experiencing clear flashes of sight.

I love life; therefore, my vision of life is clear.

It is safe for me to see.

I forgive myself, and my vision is now clear.

My negative patterns of seeing are dissolving.

My vision is perfect as I observe my perfection.

I nourish myself with healthy foods and exercise.

I love my body, my eyes, and my vision.

It is easy for me to recover my vision.

I am dealing with the tension that blurs my vision.

I am removing the obstructions to seeing the beauty of the world.

I see the wisdom and truth in life.

I am in touch with my inner desire to see.

I am working through the barriers of ignorance, fear, and anger so that my perfect vision can be realized.

I am thankful that my vision is healthy and clear.

I see things in the world that please me.

My glasses are becoming less a part of me.

I am letting healthy, alive, and creative vision manifest itself.

I am projecting my new consciousness through my eyes.

My evening vision is as clear as my daytime vision.

I see more colors with my natural vision.

As I enjoy my body, my vision becomes clearer.

As my mind becomes clear and balanced, I see more.

I am magnificent, and I am empowering myself and others with love, light, and vision.

Relaxation

An integral part of the program is to train your mind and body to relax via suggestions. Trained patients have been able to induce relaxation by talking to their body parts. In the beginning, as with any new training program, introduce specific suggestions slowly. The eyes, especially, can quickly learn to relax.

One way to relax your body is to listen to soothing music. Your choice of music could span quiet jazz, baroque, classical, or piano, flute, harp, and electronic keyboard varieties. The key is to unwind the mind, which in turn will relax the body and many of the physiological processes, including the heartbeat and the breathing.

Ultimately the eyes and the process of vision will be facilitated by this relaxation. The goal is to reach the point where you can induce a relaxed state at will during stressful periods of the day.

While researching this program, I wrote a narrative that was later turned into a "Relax and See" audiotape. To simulate the male/female association for the right and left eyes, I used two voices. My voice leads the listener on a relaxing journey, while a female voice states visually related affirmations.

The effects of the tape, measured during clinical testing, were dramatic. Most of the subjects were unable to complete the twenty-six-minute tape because they inevitably fell asleep. On average, patients fell asleep twelve minutes after the tape began. They also reported a profound overall feeling of body, mind, and eye relaxation as well as dreaming in vivid pictures. This evidence supports the theory that the unconscious mind is still recording the suggestions from the tape while the listener enters the initial stages of sleep.

More recently, I have been producing custom-made audiotapes for my patients, based on their answers to an in-depth questionnaire. The results have been most encouraging. Some of my patients have given me feedback:

"Your voice is extraordinary. . . . My eyes are measurably stronger. I now see twice as far and no longer squint. . . . I look forward to my next reduced lens prescription."

"The tape has brought fast results.... My left eye is no longer blurry and tired.... I can read again without strain."

Listening to the taped suggestions regularly during the three-phase program will create a habit of relaxing. Of course, the benefits of feeding suggestions to the unconscious mind don't have to stop at relaxation. Prior to sleeping I use tapes or imagine specific statements in my unconscious mind. Such a statement may be a form of acknowledgment, a thought to dream about, or an answer I seek to a specific challenge in my life.

Eating

You're going to be asking a lot from your eyes in the months ahead, so you'll want to nourish them with foods that will contribute to your natural vision-fitness. Set up an eating plan, and stick to it. (For some guidelines, see chapter 6.)

In case you slip and succumb to a "forbidden" food, and even if you don't slip at all, use the biofeedback from your eyes to monitor how various foods affect your vision-fitness. With every food you eat, you can experiment to learn more about your own body's needs. If you would like to follow the same diet I prescribed for the research subjects, it follows.

Foods and Substances That Patients Refrained from Eating During the Program

Alcoholic beverages	Eggs
Caffeinated foods and drinks	Fried foods
Caffeinated tea	Fruit
Canned food	Fruit juices
Cheese	Ice cream
Cigarettes	Milk
Coffee	Red meat
Drugs (unless under medical direction)	Sugared items

Preferred Foods for the Program

One salad per day

Raw/steamed/lightly cooked vegetables every day

Herb (chamomile) or bancha (twig) tea

Fasting for a day, which might involve drinking only water or vegetable juices, or fruit juices during the summer (consult your doctor before fasting)

Seasoning as recommended in macrobiotic cookbooks (see Suggested Reading)

One serving of fish or poultry every other day instead of red meat (if you are vegetarian, use bean derivatives)

Tofu (bean curd)/mochi (sweet rice)/tempeh (from soybeans)

Grains such as short-grain brown rice, millet, quinoa (Incan grain), kasha (buckwheat groats), basmati rice (long-grain Indian variety)

Root vegetables and squashes

Specific therapeutic supplementation (see Vision-Improvement Programs and Services)

Exercise

As you may recall from chapter 6, exercising your body will increase the efficiency with which the blood circulates nutrients to your eyes.

I have my patients select one or more movement or exercise activity to engage in during the three phases. Here are some suggestions:

Aerobics	Raquetball
Backpacking	Riding an exercise bike
Cycling	Rowing
Fast dancing	Skating
Jogging	Skiing

Slow dancing	Walking
Swimming	Weight lifting
Tai chi	Windsurfing
Tennis	Yoga

Natural Light

Most books on the anatomy of the eye mention that 25 percent of the visual fibers which leave the retina bypass the pathways to the visual area of the brain. It has been proposed that these fibers, carrying the electrical equivalent of white sunlight, go to a part of the brain known as the hypothalamus. This "master regulator" makes adjustments to the nervous system of the body, balancing the functions of organs such as the pituitary and adrenal glands. Also, a pea-sized organ known as the pineal gland, thought to be our primitive eye, or "third eye," is apparently "charged" by the full-spectrum white light traversing the hypothalamus. This charge may also have some influence on the balance in the nervous system, which is thought to affect our mood states and the accuracy of our perceptions.

It appears that natural, full-spectrum white sunlight keeps the bodily functions working at a minimal physiological level. In the absence of full-spectrum light, the autonomic nervous system has to make an internal adjustment. This adjustment can manifest as fatigue, a desire to eat "culprit foods," irritability, and mood shifts. To maintain the optimum balance in the nervous system, it is necessary for you to spend twenty to thirty minutes per day out of doors *without* eye devices that block natural sunlight, such as sunglasses, prescription eyeglasses, or contacts.

If the weather is pleasant, practice the vision games outside. In order to avoid unnecessary eyestrain and damage to the fovea, remember not to look directly at the sun and not to allow harsh sunlight to reflect off reading material. When you expose your eyes to natural sunlight, do so before 10:00 A.M. or after 4:00 P.M. to avoid the hottest periods of sunlight and to prevent unnecessary exposure to ultraviolet rays.

Color

Within the full spectrum of white light are all the colors of the rainbow—violet, indigo, blue, green, yellow, orange, and red. Syntonics, a branch of optometry, has been demonstrating for the past eighty years how the combination of these colors can heal various eye conditions. Other reports suggest that imaging and breathing imagined colors can have beneficial healing effects on tissues and structures of the eye. The key to this, and to all healing, is repetitive application of the technique.

Yellow, orange, and red are warming and stimulating colors. The flow of blood to the eye is activated by visualizing these colors striking the retina. Green is a harmonizing and balancing color, which is why you feel so good going for a walk in a forest or being near lush green vegetation. Blue, violet, and magenta are relaxing colors. These colors stimulate the relaxing parasympathetic branch of the autonomic nervous system, which de-stresses your nervous system, and you feel and see better. Remember that the iris muscle, which controls the size of the pupil, and the ciliary/focusing muscle are influenced by this nervous system. Relaxing colors recalibrate the nervous system so that your muscles don't become as strained and fatigued.

Spend time outdoors looking at the colors in nature. Walk through a garden. Pick vegetables of different colors and imagine the colors and nutrients increasing the well-being of your eye structures while you eat them. Using color is one way to develop a lifestyle that supports the unfolding of your clear vision.

Patches

You will use two kinds of patches during the initial two phases.

Phase One: One-Eyed Patch

During the first phase, cover your preferred eye (the eye you would sight with if you were looking through a telescope). If you wish to wear your eyeglasses, you may place a piece of paper behind one of the lenses to act as a patch.

Try to wear the patch for four continuous hours per day. In the beginning you might find it helpful to set up a wearing schedule that gradually increases. Decide what works for you according to your schedule and unique level of vision-fitness.

The four-hour patch-wearing stretch may include activities such as cooking, physical exercise (in a safe environment), watching television, doing laundry, reading, working at a desk or on a computer, taking a walk in a park, talking with friends, and so on. You could also include the time you are playing the vision games as part of the four hours. (Refer to game instructions for specific instructions on patch-wearing.) Never wear the patch while driving.

The one-eyed patch will stimulate perceptions and memories. You might have physical or even emotional responses. Record these experiences on your "Clearer Vision Phase Goals" form (see pages 101–2). If you cover your right eye, observe whether or not your speech patterns change. If you cover your left eye, notice whether it is more difficult to hear or listen to what others are saying. Connect the right-brain/left-brain aspects discussed earlier. You might notice that you don't complete tasks as quickly as usual while wearing the patch. You will be learning how to negotiate the blur. This is a very important part of the training process. Many of my patients are thankful to slow down and "see" more of life.

When your time is up, remove the patch very slowly. What happens when you remove the patch after an extended wearing period? Does your physical or emotional balance change? Enjoy the light when the patch comes off.

By the way, I encourage my patients to place stickers on their patches. If they go "public," others will want to know what is going on! By going public while working on my own vision, I learned a lot when I shared with others. Of course, you can choose to be in the closet about your patch wearing.

Phase Two: Two-Eyed Patch

During the second phase, you will put aside the one-eyed patch and will wear a two-eyed patch instead. This can be done successfully only when the difference in vision-fitness between the right and left eye is no more than 14 percent. In other words, you should be seeing equally well out of both eyes before you begin to wear the two-eyed patch. If you have a lazy eye, or an eye that turns in, you can begin wearing the two-eyed patch sooner. This new patch is designed to enhance your awareness of peripheral vision and to foster greater clarity of sight without corrective lenses.

To make the two-eyed patch, cut out a three-inch by one-inch strip of stiff cardboard. Remove a triangular piece to accommodate your nose. You can also use adhesive tape to attach the patch to your vision-fitness lenses.

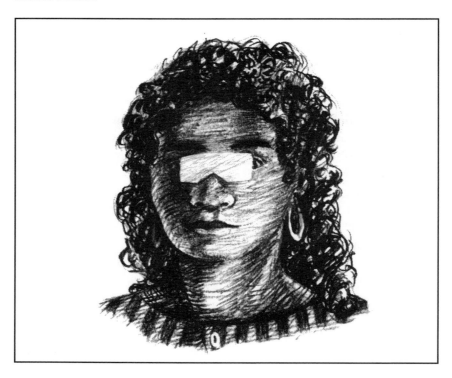

Wear your two-eyed patch instead of corrective lenses for four consecutive hours a day during Phase Two. (Wear your patch only in non-life-threatening situations.) Once again, the wearing period can include your game-playing time; refer to individual game instructions for specific guidelines on patch-wearing. In addition to playing this phase's new games, you will be repeating the games you learned in Phase One, this time while wearing the two-eyed patch.

Be sure to experiment with the new patch. Rotate your head left and right, and notice whether you perceive more easily or clearly through one side or the other. Does this correspond to your preferred eye? Now, move your head so that you perceive more out of the other, non-preferred eye, in order to develop its vision-fitness. Notice how you feel while wearing the two-eyed patch. Do you feel especially tense or relaxed? Whatever you feel while wearing the patch, see if you can re-create that sensation when not wearing the patch.

Don't hesitate to decorate your patch and venture with it into public places. Be brave. People will be genuinely interested in hearing about your program, and you might make some new friends.

Phase Three: Either Patch

During Phase Three, in order to strengthen the ability of your eyes to work together, do not wear either patch while playing the vision games. But do continue to wear either the one-eyed or the two-eyed patch every day for four continuous hours.

Vision Games

The vision-fitness exercises, which I call vision games, are distributed over the three phases, which will take between one month and two years. I like to describe the vision work as a game so that you have fun incorporating the play into your daily life.

There are new games or activities for each phase. Each vision game calls for a higher degree of vision-fitness as you move through the program.

If you decide not to do the program in its entirety, the vision games can be practiced out of sequence. For example, if you find a game that is particularly effective for your needs, play with it and develop your vision-fitness. If you find a game too complex, go back to an earlier game and master that activity before proceeding to a higher level.

When working on Activity 2, repeat Activity 1, and so on. This means that when you are on Activity 11, you'll do that activity and repeat all the previous activities. You will be working toward mastery of each activity and developing your vision-fitness in a systematic way.

Once you have completed Phase One, repeat the Phase One games while wearing the two-eyed patch, and also begin the Phase Two games. Both eyes will have a chance to increase their vision-fitness by playing the one-eyed games while wearing the two-eyed patch.

In Phase Three, repeat the Phase One and the Phase Two games with both eyes open. During this phase you will train the cells in the brain that respond to two-eyed activity. Don't forget to still wear either the one-eyed patch or the two-eyed patch for four continuous hours often during Phase Three.

In all the phases, remember to remove your contacts and/or eyeglasses during the vision games. (In some cases, you might experiment using your reduced-power prescription.) Read the instructions for each activity, and reread them when you play the vision game. Also, set aside a specific time for your vision games on your "Clearer Vision Phase Goals" form, recognizing that Phases Two and Three will require more time to play.

Notice that I make specific mention of those vision games that are helpful for dyslexia, reading problems, eye "dis-ease," computer work and other causes of eyestrain, farsightedness, nearsightedness, and astigmatism. Many patients choose individual games from the program that can help them overcome particular vision challenges. The following summary indicates games that are helpful for overcoming specific challenges.

Vision Games for Specific Vision Challenges

Farsightedness: Zooming, Near Eye-C chart, lighting, fencing

Nearsightedness: Distance Eye-C chart, soft focus, imaging, painting

Astigmatism: Painting, palming, eye-muscle stretch, fencing

Eye "dis-ease": Imaging, acupressure, yawning, palming

Computer-related eyestrain: Zooming, Eye-C chart, shifting, palming

Dyslexia: Marching, swing ball, string thing, fencing

Slow reading: String thing, fencing, finger doubling, circles

Children's vision: Palming, swing ball, fencing, lighting, eye-muscle stretch, marching

Recordkeeping

Review your overall goals at the transition point from one phase to the next. Each day complete the "Results produced" section, Eye-C chart measurements, and the "Physical and emotional responses" section of the "Clearer Vision Phase Goals" form. Choose your affirmations and goals for the next day, and the times you plan to implement the goals. When you complete the program, you will have a diary of your adventures.

Clearer Vision Phase Goals

Phase _____ Activity _____

Affirmation _____

Goals

Implementation time
Goal #

1 _____ _____ 7 A.M. _____ 5 P.M.

2 _____ _____ 8 A.M. _____ 6 P.M.

3 _____ _____ 9 A.M. _____ 7 P.M.

4 _____ _____ 10 A.M. _____ 8 P.M.

5 _____ _____ 11 A.M. _____ 9 P.M.

6 _____ _____ noon _____ 10 P.M.

7 _____ _____ 1 P.M. _____ 11 P.M.

8 _____ _____ 2 P.M.

9 _____ _____ 3 P.M.

10 _____ _____ 4 P.M.

Notes _____

_____

_____

_____

_____

_____

Results produced

1 _____
2 _____
3 _____
4 _____
5 _____
6 _____
7 _____

		Far	Near
Eye-C Chart	Right	_____	_____
	Left	_____	_____
	Both	_____	_____

Physical and emotional responses _____

_____
_____
_____
_____
_____
_____
_____

Phase One

Phase One, Activity 1: Zooming

Purpose   To train flexible focus between your mind and your eyes.

Materials   Your thumb, an eraser, a window, a person's face, or any nearby object that is at a distance between your eyes and farther objects.

Instructions Zooming means to shift your focus quickly from a near distance to a far distance. For example, imagine looking from a nearby red flower to a distant forest.

Wearing your one-eyed patch, sit comfortably in a chair and position your thumb or index finger in front of your non-patched eye.

Take a deep breath, and imagine air flowing into your eyes. (You can use this type of breathing with all the vision games.)

While looking at your finger, notice how blurry everything is beyond the finger. "See" to the right, left, up, and down while you continue to look at the finger.

The more you are aware of the blur, the clearer the thumb will appear. This awareness is helpful for improving fitness of your foveal eyesight. Let the blur represent your awareness of your retina.

Now move your focus of attention toward an object farther from your thumb. Repeat to farther and farther distances. Repeat the exercise, changing your focus back and forth from a near to a distant object.

Now walk around the room you're in and see everything while looking at either your finger or a distant point.

Think of the blur as a connection to your past vision. See beyond your limiting filters of the past. Dissolve the memory implant that says you can't see. As you zoom back and forth, experience your vision free of the belief filters of the past. Imagine that your brain and eyes have the internal knowledge to produce self-healing.

Zoom and see now as an observer with little or no thinking. Rather than thinking, feel what you see. Zooming allows you to move out into your visual world through the blur.

Repeat the zooming for ten to twenty breaths three times during the day.

Keeping your head still, use your eyes to track the motion of your finger as you move it in a horizontal arc. Notice the motion of the objects behind your finger.

Observations   Are you staring, holding your breath, or not blinking?

Do you have any physical reactions such as tension in the stomach, shoulders, neck, or behind the head?

How safe do you feel as you reach out into the blur?

Do you experience any feelings of sadness, happiness, joy, terror, nervousness, loneliness, or anxiety?

Do you feel an urge to rip off the patch?

Phase One, Activity 2: Palming

Purpose   To use your healing hands to direct specific energy and images toward and away from your eyes.

Materials   A pillow and your hands.

Instructions   Make yourself comfortable by resting your elbows on a table or placing a pillow on your chest to rest your arms.

Gently rub your palms together, generating warmth.

Place your warm palms over your relaxed, closed eyelids. The palms should not be pressed against the eyes but should gently rest on the bony ridge surrounding the eyes.

Imagine that your palms are like magnets that draw tension away from the eyelids and the muscles of your eyes.

During the colder months, visualize the warmth as a down comforter or a sleeping bag that is warming the structures of your eyes.

Visualize the different parts of the eyes relaxing the way your body muscles let go in a hot bath.

Feel the warmth from your palms as you breathe.

Imagine, with each breath, healthy blood flowing from the heart, up the spine, into your brain, down the optic nerve, and into your eyes.

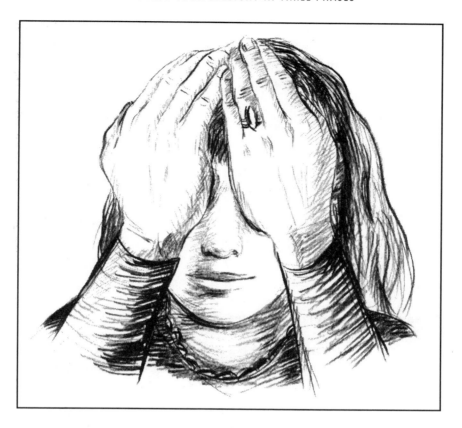

Picture the healthy blood carrying oxygen and nutrients from the healthy foods you are eating. Let the vitamins and minerals flow to the eye structures: vitamin A and zinc to the retina; B-complex to the macula and fovea; chromium to the focusing muscle; and vitamins C, E, and B_2 to the lens, which remolds to a perfect shape for 20/20 vision.

Palm for a minimum of two minutes, two or three times per day. You can palm for as long as fifteen minutes and use this as your daily relaxation exercise.

You can also use the number of breaths you take as a way to program how long to palm. It takes between two and three minutes to breath thirty times.

Observations   Can you produce a color sensation of deep blue or violet while palming? Is there a relationship between thinking and your ability to see dark color?

Does your mind or inner voice interfere with this vision game?

Can you slow down your breathing while you palm your eyes?

How do you feel about your blur when you remove your palms?

Do you notice how bright everything looks?

Do objects appear clearer?

When your eyes open, can you pretend you have full use of your vision?

Be ready to have clear flashes of perfect sight.

Reminder   Remember to repeat the vision game in Activity 1.

Phase One, Activity 3: Eye-C Chart

Purpose   To observe and become aware of the way relaxation, mind strain, affirmations, foods, stress, and light affect your perceptions on a simulated eye chart.

Materials   Have a copy made of the two Eye-C charts, or remove them from the book. Place the larger Distance Eye-C chart on a wall five feet away. The smaller Near Eye-C chart should be placed approximately sixteen inches from your eyes.

Instructions   If your challenge is seeing things far away, begin with the Distance Eye-C chart. If things up close are blurry, begin with the Near Eye-C chart.

Distance chart   Make sure there is enough light shining on the chart. Use a 100-watt daylight-blue color-corrected or full-spectrum light bulb (see Vision-Improvement Programs and Services) shining from a three-foot distance.

Stand or sit between five and twenty feet from the chart. Choose a distance at which you can just make out the letters in the middle of the chart. Patch your preferred eye, and see which letters on the Eye-C chart are clear enough for you to make out.

This is not a test. You are training yourself to be relaxed in front of a simulated eye chart. This awareness will allow you to be more comfortable and skilled when you go back to your eye doctor to have your vision measured. If you can train yourself to be comfortable, confident, and relaxed with the Eye-C chart, the regular Snellen chart will be easier to perceive. Your eye doctor's measurements will then be made under more relaxed conditions.

E	9
B C	8
F D L	7
P T E O	6
Z B F D E	5
L C T B F O	4
P E O F D L Z	3
O Z B T D F C E	2
B L D E C Z O P F	1

E 100

B C 50

F D L 35

P T E O 25

Z B F D E 20

L C T B F O 15

P E O F D L Z 10

O Z B T D F C E 7.5

B L D E C Z O P F 5

Note the smallest line of letters that you can see. On your "Clearer Vision Phase Goals" form, record the vision-fitness number that is alongside the line of letters as well as the distance from your eyes to the chart. If you like, you may also verify how the patched eye is perceiving.

You might have a clear transparency made of the Distance Eye-C chart and place it on a window so that you can look through the chart while still maintaining your seeing of the chart. (This will be covered in more detail in activities 15 through 19.)

Later on in the program you will learn more advanced looking and seeing strategies that can be practiced while playing the Eye-C chart game.

Near chart Use a 60- or 100-watt bulb shining on the chart from a distance of three feet.

Hold the chart at a distance equivalent to the distance from your middle knuckle to your elbow, or whatever distance allows you to clearly see some of the letters.

Cover your preferred eye with the patch. If you cannot make out any letters or words, then slip on your reduced-power lenses.

The goal of the game is to make out smaller and smaller print, letters, or words. Note the vision-fitness number on the smallest line of letters that you can make out on the Eye-C chart. Move the chart back and forth and see if through relaxation you can keep the letters clear as you bring the chart closer to your eyes. Spend about five minutes playing with the Eye-C chart.

Make extra copies to place in different parts of your home or office. As you walk by the Eye-C chart, glance at it and check your ability to perceive. In this way you can begin using your eyes as the biofeedback device discussed in chapter 3.

When there is a great variation, begin looking for the cause of the change.

Observations   While playing with the Eye-C charts, begin to incorporate earlier games such as zooming, palming, breathing, and blinking.

Zoom from the Distance Eye-C chart to the near one and vice versa.

When using the distance chart, zoom onto your index finger or thumb at six inches from your eyes. Breathe in when you look up close and out when you zoom far away. How does it feel when you breathe? Do you experience clear flashes of the letters?

Imagine white light rather than letters emanating from the Eye-C charts. Absorb and receive this white light with no expectation about the clarity of the letters.

The idea is to let go of trying to make the letters clear. The flashes of clarity will happen on their own; you do not have to try to make this happen. Trying actually defeats the purpose of clearer vision. Trying harder is a cultural bad habit that many of us have imprinted into our belief system.

Phase One, Activity 4: Soft Focus

Purpose   To train yourself to look in a relaxed way while seeing.

Materials   The Distance or Near Eye-C charts or any other object that has a lot of detail.

Instructions   As in zooming, when you practice soft focus, try to become aware of the object or detail you are looking at. Let the point of focus (object) represent your fovea in space. Let the area around the looking point (background) be the retina in space. As long as you are looking and seeing simultaneously, you will be simulating a soft focus.

Unlike the earlier activities, soft focus can be done for short periods of non-blinking, from five to twenty-five seconds. Usually a lack of blinking implies that you're staring. But if you follow the directions above, no harm will result by delaying your blinking. I have seen patients go without blinking for sixty seconds and longer while soft-focusing. Observe whether or not blinking pulls your vision closer toward the clearer zone of seeing. Systematic diaphragm breathing is the important variable. As long as the breath is flowing, you will be in soft focus rather than staring.

Soft focus can be played while you read, work at a computer terminal, or play sports.

If you are wearing your regular strong eyeglasses, you can use soft focus to prevent staring. While soft-focusing, imagine that you are moving out into your visual world, as if you are looking through the blur.

Soft focus for five minutes every day.

Observations   In the beginning, catch yourself when you are not soft-focusing, and then move into soft-focusing.

Can you soft focus while working at your job, cooking, cleaning house, going for a walk, or watching television?

Do you feel more balanced when you soft focus? Begin soft-focusing on the parts of yourself you may not have wished to see. These may have to do with hidden talents, the desire for a new job or a different relationship, or friends and family whom you have neglected.

Phase One, Activity 5: Painting/Yawning

Purpose   To teach the mind's eye to see white, to release tension in the muscles of the face and jaw, and to produce flowing tears, which will bathe and soothe the cornea.

Instructions   Begin with yawning. Granted, it is considered to be bad manners in our culture to yawn. For this game, however, you have permission to yawn freely, and I am talking about a loud animal yawn where the jaws are wide open and you expel sounds through your mouth. To release your inhibitions, imagine that you are visiting a zoo and are playing with the chimpanzees. Let go of all the holds you have on expressing animal sounds. Let others around you know about the game you are playing.

Play the yawning game until tears flow down your cheeks. When you produce tears, imagine that the toxins within your eyes are flowing away and healthy nutrients are flowing in. After a while, you will probably find the yawning game to be relaxing, and the flashes of clear vision will occur more frequently.

Now that you feel relaxed and more present, close your eyes and imagine that a paintbrush is attached to

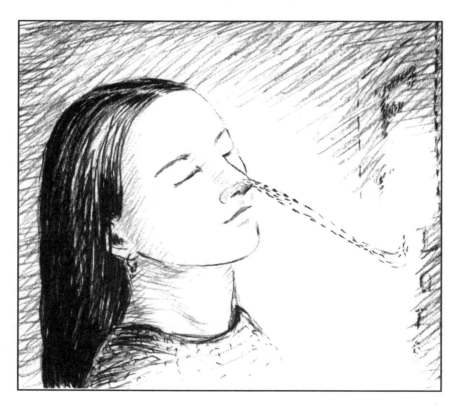

the end of your nose. You can paint anything you want by moving your head.

In the beginning, imagine that the only paint you have is white, and as a game, you are going to paint everything in sight white. You can begin with your bedroom, then the living room, the rest of your home, and your place of work. Enjoy seeing everything as white in your mind's eye.

Imagine painting the Eye-C chart so that all the letters are covered. Experience in your mind's eye seeing the white light beaming off the chart and coming into your eyes and into your "third eye" (between your eyes on your forehead).

Give a few more yawns to help you see the whiteness. Spend five to ten minutes playing these two games.

Painting teaches you to enjoy white, which is the light emitted by the sun with all the colors present. This game is also designed to familiarize you with the idea of being able to see white. As you will experience in Phase Two, white light can be used for self-healing.

Find several times during the day when you can yawn or paint. If you travel on a bus or by train, close your eyes, image the persons around you, and paint them white. When you are waiting at stoplights, give a mighty yawn. Grade yourself on the intensity of the yawns.

Observations   Sit in front of the Eye-C chart. After a yawning spell and two or three minutes painting white, look again at the letters on the chart. Are you able to see more, or less, clearly? Are you able to relax your mind during this vision game?

Talk to your brain and let it know that you would like to see more clearly as quickly as possible.

Phase One, Activity 6: Swing Ball

Purpose   To activate and integrate all the parts of the brain into synchronous whole-brain perceptions.

Materials

Obtain a soft, colored ball about three inches in diameter. Attach a ten-foot string to the ball by bending a large paper clip and pushing it through the ball.

Attach the string to a hook in the ceiling. Adjust the length of the string so that when you are lying underneath the ball, it is about sixteen inches from your eyes.

Reminder

Remember to use the one-eyed patch during Phase One, the two-eyed patch during Phase Two, and no patch during Phase Three.

Instructions

Lie underneath the ball on a comfortable surface such as a carpet, mat, or bed. Make sure that your entire body is relaxed.

Place your head so that the ball is directly in front of your uncovered eye or eyes. Look at the ball and see all the other areas of space around the ball. Let your vision wander around the room while you look at the ball. (Remember, your fovea is represented by the ball, and your retina is the rest of the space.)

Follow the same directions as in zooming and the other vision games you have been mastering. Breathe as you zoom from the ball to the ceiling. Imagine more and more areas of space coming into focus.

This phase of swing ball is mastered without the influence of gravity. Later you will repeat the same game while standing.

You may wish to place an Eye-C chart on the ceiling where the string is attached in order to observe changes in visual clarity as you play the swing-ball game.

Gently push the ball so that it begins to swing from above your head toward your feet. Use baroque music to create rhythm for the game. I like Vivaldi's *Four Seasons*.

Tune in to your breathing as you train your eyes to follow the swinging ball. The goal is to keep your mind and eyes free of strain.

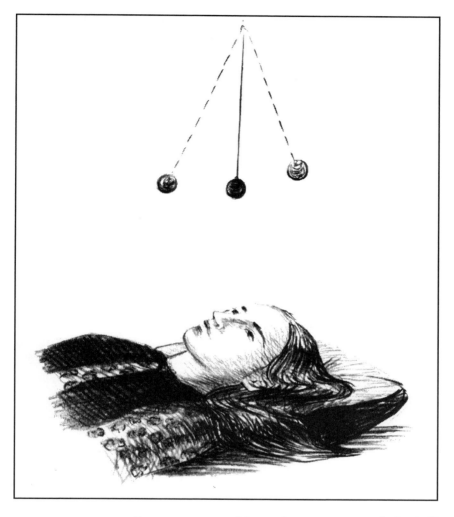

Become aware of how the space around the ball seems to be moving really fast. This is like being on a fast-moving train and looking out the window, watching the nearby scenery zooming by.

You might feel squeezing or warm sensations in your stomach or chest area. Repeat this phase until your body and mind feel more relaxed.

You will learn to feel your body and emotions more profoundly than usual during the swing-ball game. I believe that the up-and-down motion of the ball affects the *chakras*, the seven energy centers of the body. According to this theory, as you follow the ball, the motion of your eyes directs a flow of energy to the center corresponding to the position of the ball. For example, when the ball is positioned over the heart area, the eyes are looking in that direction, and the energy center associated with the heart chakra is then stimulated. My personal experience is that I feel more connection between my body, mind, spirit, and eyes after five minutes of this phase of swing ball.

For the next phase, follow the ball as it swings left and right across your uncovered eye(s), maintaining the same sixteen-inch distance. The left and right movement of your eyes will help to synchronize the brain hemispheres. Research has shown that when your eyes look to the left, you stimulate the right hemisphere, and vice versa. Crossing over at the midline of the eyes leads to a powerful "switching" that promotes the integration process within the brain.

Many patients who experience motion sickness have been helped by this exercise. I remember a dyslexic patient saying at this point in the game, "I think my eye is drunk!"

Repeat for twenty to fifty breaths. You should feel your eyes moving very smoothly during the left-to-right movement. Let the swing ball set the rhythm for your breathing.

Occasionally, zoom to the ceiling and then back to the ball. How quickly can you change focus?

When you have mastery, add another variable. Now when the ball goes to the right, say "right," and when the ball goes to the left, say "left." Repeat until you feel total flow, and trust that you can play the game effortlessly .

Now say the opposite. Call out "left" when the ball swings to the right, and "right" when the ball swings to the left.

When you've mastered that, lift your left arm when your eyes go to the left and you say "right," and vice versa. As you can see, the game can become quite complex and require a lot of memory, trust, and vision, but remember, what you can remember, you can see.

When you are ready for another challenge, choose a word to spell. When the ball goes to the left, without moving your arms, say the first letter. Say the second letter when the ball goes to the right.

Pay attention to the movement of your eyes rather than to your head. I notice that when patients begin thinking about the word, as opposed to picturing the word, their eyes tend to stop moving.

When your vision-fitness at this level is developed, include arm and even leg movements with the spelling.

Finally, choose two words. Spell one of the words on the right side while you spell the other word on the left side. If the two words were *Texas* and *Oregon*, you would start off by designating *Texas* to the left and *Oregon* to the right. When the ball swings to the right, you would spell *O*, then follow the ball to the left and spell *T*, and on. This calls for high degrees of visual imagery, memory, sequencing, and visual attention.

Later, you can introduce right-arm and left-leg movements while you spell. Again, relaxing music can be used, or you could eventually use rock music as a distractor.

The goal is to be able to play the swing-ball game while spelling, moving the assigned body parts, and listening to potentially distracting music. When you can do all of this easily, repeat the whole process while standing with the swing ball at eye level. At this point your vision and your brain will be well synchronized, and your vision process will be in its most relaxed mode.

Observations   Are you aware of your surroundings while following the ball and playing the rest of the game?

Are you able to relax so that each new level is viewed as a challenge and you master it quickly?

Do you feel dizzy, nauseous, or disoriented?

If your vision-fitness is at a level where you decide to stay at one phase of the swing-ball game, do not feel that you have to master the next level right away. You have the rest of your life to master the higher levels.

Feel free to repeat earlier vision games at any point in the sequence. Let your eyes tell you when to take a break. For example, if you feel frustrated during the swing-ball game, take off your patch and palm your eyes. Notice whether this brings you back to the point where you feel relaxed enough to continue.

Finally, you can transfer this new awareness into your daily life. If you experience "blocks" in your ability to visually process while working on a particular project, or if the blur begins to influence your productivity or behavior, then put one or more of the vision games into action. By the end of the three phases, vision-fitness will be a fully integrated part of your daily routine, and you will have mastered a set of new skills.

Phase One, Activity 7: Shifting/Scanning

Purpose   To heighten your awareness that eye movement leads to more relaxed and broader perception.

Instructions   This is the last vision game you will play using the one-eyed patch. Use the Eye-C chart, a book, a friend's face, the view from a window, or a television.

Choose two points, one in the left, the other in the right part of your visual field. Let your eye shift back and forth between the two points as you breathe. Also add palming, soft focus, and zooming.

Feel what it is like to have the eye move in a relaxed way without any strain. This game will allow you to break any habitual patterns of staring or straining. Continue shifting between the points for twenty breaths.

If you use someone's face, shift from earlobe to eyebrow, chin, nose, eye, cheek, and so on. This shifting is particularly helpful if you work at a computer. Shift between points on the screen while the computer is accessing data.

Computer users can place an Eye-C chart on a wall or a window beyond or alongside their workstations. Zooming your eyes from the computer screen to the Eye-C chart will allow you to verify that your Eye-C vision-fitness is maintained. If the chart starts to look more blurry, spend some time palming.

The next phase is to introduce scanning, or painting with the eyes open. Scanning is moving the eyes as in painting, but without the imaginary paintbrush. Use the earlier painting game and begin scanning along the Eye-C chart, your friend's face, paintings, scenes out a window, the computer screen, or even your book.

Unlike shifting, scanning is soft and gentle. In the beginning, you might find yourself holding your breath. The goal is to develop flow and ease while scanning.

Combine the feeling you mastered in soft focus and the awareness you developed from swing ball when shifting and scanning.

Repeat for five minutes per day, or play two or three times during the day for shorter periods. As with other games, you may spend as much time as you like on this game while mastering it.

Observations Watch for shallow breathing and trying too hard. Observe your posture. I have noticed that my patients tend to lean forward during this game.

Can you incorporate the awareness gained from shifting/scanning into your daily life? Try using this game while standing in line, at the stoplight, on the train or bus, and while cooking, cleaning your house, and shaving or putting on makeup.

How is your performance on the Eye-C chart while you shift from the right side of the chart to the left?

Do you appreciate more details if you gently scan each row of letters, paint them white, and allow the whiteness to come to your eyes?

Shift from one row of letters to another.

Because letter charts ask you to perceive in two dimensions, you might begin to strain. Balanced vision occurs when you see in three dimensions, so try to see the three-dimensionality of the Eye-C chart.

If your eyes are not moving, begin shifting and scanning.

Phase Two

Phase Two, Activity 8: Nose Pencil

Purpose To transfer the awareness of painting with the eyes closed into your open-eyed visual world.

Instructions Wearing your two-eyed patch, spend a few minutes walking around, adjusting to this new way of perceiving.

Notice whether you tend to look more out of one eye than both. If so, is it your preferred eye, which was covered during Phase One?

Adjust your head, if necessary, so that you are looking out of your non-preferred eye. Now you can choose which eye to look out of under different conditions.

You might find it overly challenging to look through both eyes while doing book or desk work with the two-eyed patch in place. If so, look out of the non-preferred eye, and later, do activities that permit you to peep out of both eyes. You could also make another two-eyed patch that is 1.5 millimeters shorter on each side to use for reading. You will find it easier to look out of both eyes with the narrower two-eyed patch.

The goal is to see a little out of the right eye and a little out of the left. If you align your head in exactly the right position, your sight will increase.

Now recall the paintbrush on the end of your nose. Conjure up an image of painting a picture white. I like to paint any unpleasant picture white. When the picture is completely white, I imagine a pencil on the end of my nose. I open my eyes and pretend that the pencil can be any color. I then look at a blank wall and paint a new, pleasant picture. Then I sketch the corners of the room, objects seen through the window, and furniture or items on the walls. The goal is to train your mind's eye to lead your physical eye. Repeat the nose-pencil game for five minutes per day.

Observations   Can you zoom to different distances and use the nose pencil?

Notice any strain or tension that may appear in the eyes or the muscles around them.

Introduce soft focus between sessions of the nose-pencil game. Shift and scan using the nose pencil.

Are certain things more difficult than others to sketch with the nose pencil?

Do you favor looking through one eye more than the other? Can you maintain looking through both eyes?

Phase Two, Activity 9: Lighting

Purpose To train your eyes and brain to enjoy light, and to allow the light rays to heal your eyes.

Materials Ideally, you would use the sun for this game, but in many parts of the world the sun is available only during certain periods of the year—and under no circumstances should you look directly at the sun. The next-best light source is a 60- or 100-watt daylight-blue color-corrected incandescent bulb (see Vision-Improvement Programs and Services). Using this bulb, the lighting vision game can be played inside.

Make sure to place the bulb in a desk lamp which has a funnel shade so that you are not looking directly into the bulb when you are working.

Instructions Stand or sit comfortably. Close your eyes and aim them toward the sun or the light bulb.

The two-eyed patch will block some of the rays, but the outer part of your eyes will feel the warmth.

While you are appreciating the warmth, imagine the white rays of light beaming down toward you. Imagine yourself being transparent, and let the rays come to you. Picture all the colors of the spectrum: violet, indigo, blue, green, yellow, orange, and red.

Absorb the light and convert it to pictures of what you wish to see. (Recall your purpose and goals.) Let your eyes move slightly behind your closed lids. Now take an imaginary journey to the coast on a warm sunny day.

Move your head to the left and then to the right so that each (closed) eye receives exposure to the light through the eyelid.

Imagine your "third eye" opening wide, like a flower slowly opening its bud, as you are receiving all the wavelengths of light beneficial for healing your eyes.

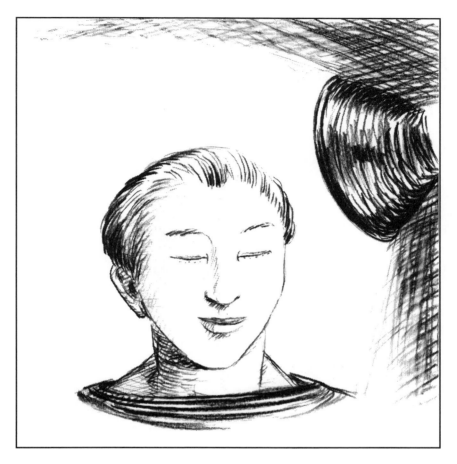

Pretend that the rays of light are traveling into your eyes and bouncing like rubber balls against your retina, stimulating the rods and cones.

Picture the little pineal gland, situated behind the third eye, receiving this healthy light. Just as a battery can be charged, let the pineal gland glow with a charge of any color you choose. Let that glow now flow outward in the form of seeing through the third eye.

As you experience the feeling of the glow, begin blinking your eyes once or twice as you rotate your head back and forth. Enjoy the light entering the eyes.

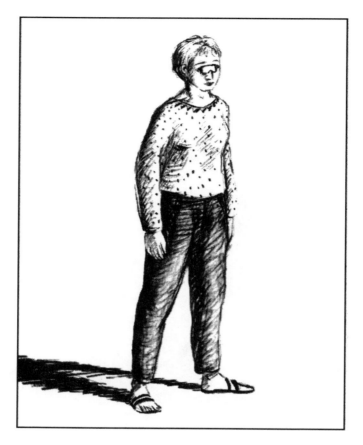

Picture your pupil shutting down and opening up as you blink. Feel the iris muscle exercising as the pupil changes size.

Repeat for fifty to 100 breaths or more per day.

If you work at a computer, use this lighting game every other hour for a minute at a time.

Also, for this phase, read with one eye while wearing the two-eyed patch. Experiment by reading with the non-preferred eye. Read a magazine or a book in candlelight that is placed thirteen to sixteen inches from your eyes.

If you notice any eyestrain, stop reading and palm or zoom. Zoom onto the patch and then far away for ten breaths. How does it feel to zoom as close as the patch? Do you feel the eye muscles pulling?

Ask your support person to check that your eyes are turning in equally.

Observations   As you master this game, you may find that your relationship with light changes. I found that I no longer grabbed for my sunglasses, particularly as I modified my intake of fatty and oily foods.

Lighting is particularly helpful for the two varieties of farsightedness. This exercise helps *presbyopia*—the farsightedness associated with age that affects your ability to read small print—by keeping the pupil small, which increases the depth of focus. The increase in contrast helps the ciliary muscle to adjust its focus. The lighting game also relaxes the strain on the focusing muscle, which is helpful for routine farsightedness.

Phase Two, Activity 10: Dynamic Visual Meditation

Purpose   To train you to be relaxed and unfocused and to visually let go while introducing body motion.

Instructions   Wear comfortable, loose clothes. While wearing the two-eyed patch for this phase, stand erect with your feet at shoulder-width apart.

With your eyes closed, begin to rotate your shoulders, hips, and head to the left; all should move together. Repeat this movement to the right, then to the left again, until you are swinging back and forth. Allow your arms to swing freely—you may find them wrapping around your body as you turn. When going to the left, let the right foot turn with the heel coming up and out like a golf swing. Repeat for the right foot when swinging to the left. In the beginning, continue in this way for ten minutes.

If you experience dizziness or fall over, check to see whether you are thinking. When you can produce

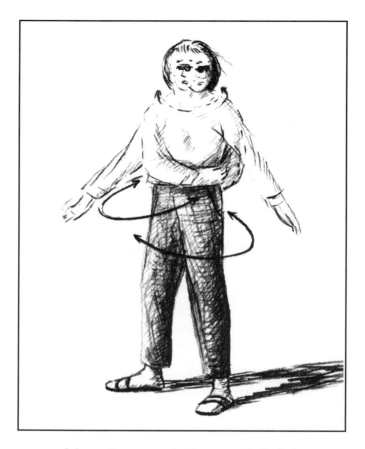

a peacefulness in your mind, you will find that your balance is perfect. Breathe, and picture forests, mountains, or the ocean. Feel your body moving in a rhythmic way. Let go of all thoughts, like leaves falling off a tree in the fall.

When you have mastered this phase, close your eyes and focus on your eyelids. Imagine that you can look out through your closed eyelids. What would you see?

Can you picture the room moving around as if you are riding a carousel horse at an amusement park? Imagine that you can perceive the world zooming by as you play the dynamic visual meditation (DVM) game.

Extend your perception even farther. Pretend that you have bionic or laser eyes and that you can see through the walls. You can see across the city, the state, the country, the planet, and into outer space.

While you do this, continue to move your body back and forth with your eyes closed.

How far can you visualize before the picture becomes foggy or blurry?

Open your eyes and continue the DVM. At first pay attention to the patch as you swing. Attempt to look through the patch as you did with your closed eyelids. Gradually begin to look around the sides of the patch.

The goal is to feel your eyes being perfectly still. Your eyes should move only in alignment with your head, shoulders, and hips.

Play the game in stages. It is important to master each stage before going on to the next.

Observations   Ask someone to watch your eyes to make sure that there are no jerky eye movements.

If you feel strain or fatigue, paint white or shift and scan for a short time.

Incorporate the games from Phase One into the DVM.

I have found the *Brandenburg Concertos* by Bach to provide a suitable tempo for this game. Experiment with different music. How does the Eye-C chart appear with the two-eyed patch after this game? What happens to your looking and seeing if you remove the patch?

Phase Two, Activity 11: Eye-Muscle Stretch

Purpose   To master stretching the eye muscles in order to relieve tension while staying relaxed.

Instructions   Wearing the two-eyed patch, seat yourself comfortably with your hands supported on your lap and your feet squarely on the floor.

Take a few deep breaths, and then, on one of the in-breaths, stretch your eyes upward. The goal is to stretch your eyes as high as they can go without straining.

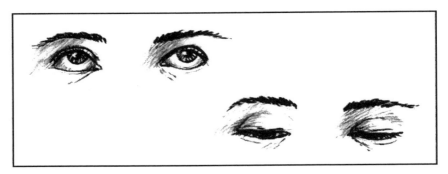

Hold your breath, and when you are ready to exhale, stretch the muscles into a downward position and breathe out. Repeat this up-and-down movement for three breaths. Then stretch to the left and right as well as up and to the left, and down and to the right. Be aware of your right visual field when you stretch to the right, and vice versa.

When you have mastered the steps above, let your eyes move around in circles. Stretch the muscles to their extremities, but don't strain them. Your eyes should feel "alive" after three to five breaths of rotations in both directions.

Remember that vision-fitness develops when the vision game is easy, without strain and tension. If you

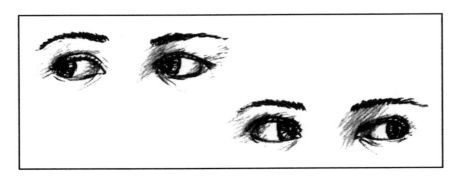

feel any tension, breathe a little more into the tight-ness. Avoid extreme stretching, as this may produce additional strain.

When you have completed all the directions, reverse the breath. Breathe out as you stretch your eyes upward.

Then remove the two-eyed patch and palm your eyes.

Repeat the eye-muscle stretch three to six times during the day. You can stretch your eyes while you exercise, cook, watch television, read, work on the computer, stand in line, or walk.

Observations   In the beginning, you may notice particular places in the muscles where there is tension. As you play the game, you will find that the tension dissipates.

Monitor your Eye-C vision-fitness after a stretch-ing session. Squeeze your eyes gently closed after stretching.

Phase Two, Activity 12: Marching

Purpose   To train your brain, eyes, and body to synchronize into whole-brain functioning.

Instructions   Stand erect with your arms at your side, shoulders back, and legs together.

Choose a point in space, preferably looking through a window. Involve both eyes, seeing around the corners of the two-eyed patch.

Begin the game by imagining that you are a soldier. Let your left leg and left arm shoot out at the same time. Then repeat for the right side. Repeat this one-sided marching for fifty breaths. March at a pace equivalent to a brisk walk, and coordinate your breathing.

When you have mastered same-side movements, move your eyes to the left when you move your left limbs, and vice versa. This may be challenging at first. Be patient and give yourself plenty of breaks.

When you have mastered this phase, begin humming a tune while you continue marching. The goal is to be involved in the game in such a relaxed way that you can let your mind wander to the beach, the forests, and the mountains, and you will not fall over.

Next, switch to a higher level: move the left arm and right leg out at the same time. This is the traditional reciprocal marching. In the beginning, let the eyes look in front again. Then add the eye movements, and finally add humming. Be brave and add spelling while marching.

Observations   I march on a small rebounder trampoline while looking through my window, watching the birds.

March in front of the Eye-C chart. Cross your eyes onto the patch and then look at the letters.

Paint white while you march.

Try to maintain your smooth marching while listening to distracting music, or have a friend attempt to distract you.

This game is particularly useful for developing vision-fitness for people with dyslexia and reading disabilities.

By now I hope you are realizing that the only limitation to having fun with the vision games is a lack of imagination.

Phase Two, Activity 13: Acupressure

Purpose   To stimulate the acupressure/acupuncture points using pressure and massage from your fingers. (Acupressure involves stimulating nerve and energy points by applying pressure with your fingers. Acupuncture is a similar process in which an acupuncturist inserts needles to accomplish the stimulation.)

Instructions   Do not wear patches for this game. Begin with the hoku point (see illustration), which is the cardinal point for the organs of the head and the eyes. Stimulating this point can relieve headaches.

Place the thumb and the index finger of the left hand together. Locate the muscular hill of the right hand. Separate the index finger and the thumb of the left hand. Place the left-hand thumb on the muscular hill. Position the left index finger on the inside of the right palm corresponding to the point of the muscular hill. Repeat the process, placing the right thumb and index finger on the muscular hill of the left hand.

Hoku point

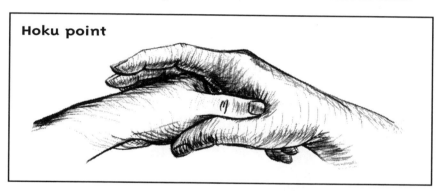

Increase the pressure of the thumb and the index finger against each other. You will be applying pressure to the hoku point. Stimulate each hand for ten to twenty breaths.

The eyebrow/thumb point has proven helpful for enhancing Eye-C performance.

Use your thumbs to massage or to apply pressure to the inside corners of your eyebrows. Add pressure to this point until the first feeling of discomfort. The other fingers can be placed on the forehead.

The nose point is stimulated by using the thumb and the index finger over the bridge of the nose. Stimulating this point relieves the pressure buildup due to straining.

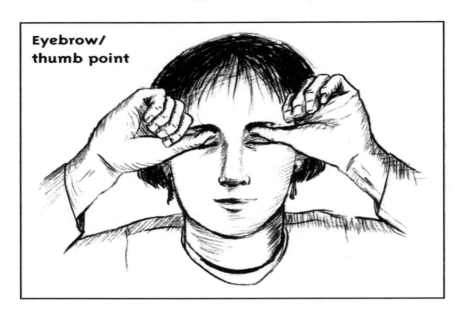

Eyebrow/
thumb point

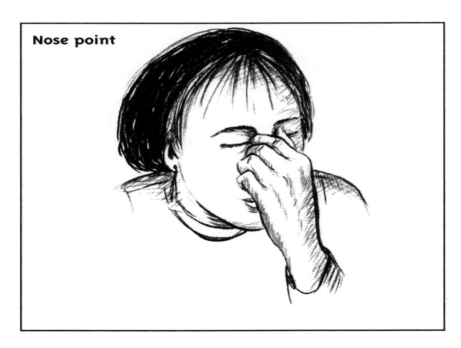

Nose point

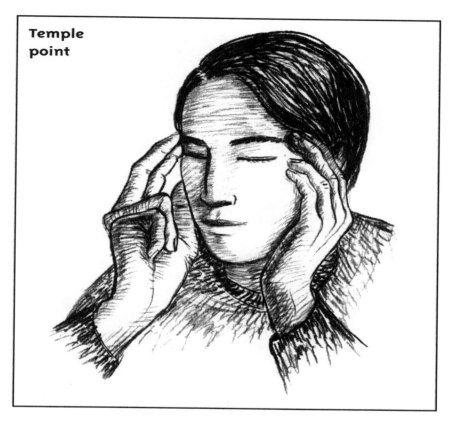

Temple point

The temple point is found in a hollow on the side of the head. Massaging this point relieves headaches or pressure in the temples. Place your index fingers on both temples and locate the hollow space. Apply pressure and massage this point for ten to twenty breaths.

Use your fingers and thumbs to massage the eyebrow and cheek points. Follow the directions in the illustration. Stimulating the eyebrow point relieves tightness due to eyestrain. Massaging the cheek point clears the sinuses and helps you to breath more easily.

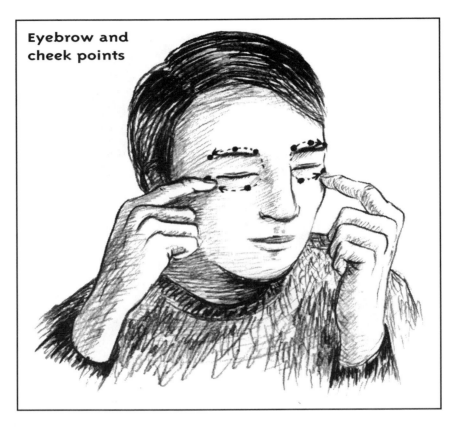

Eyebrow and cheek points

Observations   Combine the acupressure game with the Eye-C chart. How is your general disposition after the game? Find the acupressure point that is most effective in relieving tension for you.

Phase Two, Activity 14: Shoulder and Neck Massage

Purpose   To relieve tension and to improve the flow of blood to the eyes.

Instructions   Ideally, this vision game is best performed with the assistance of a support person, but you can play alone.

When you are playing on your own, place your left hand over your right shoulder. Using your four fingers, massage the shoulder muscle. Concentrate on

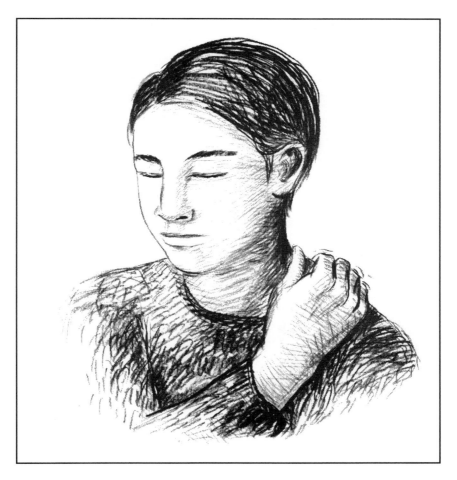

the muscle that is near the neck, and work your way toward the shoulder.

Breathe and look into the distance while performing the massage.

After a while, let your neck roll a few times, making a circle.

Repeat the same process with your right hand over your left shoulder.

An area that feels like two bumps or ridges on the back of the neck is another acupressure point related to vision, as is the back of the neck in general.

Place your thumbs on the two ridges at the back of your head. Let the rest of your fingers relax on your head. Put as much pressure on the ridges, or underneath them, as you can tolerate.

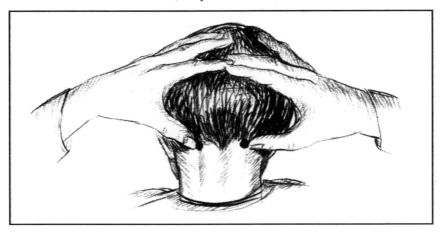

Watch the Eye-C chart and enjoy the flashes of clarity.

Repeat for twenty to fifty breaths. When you are at work, play this game for five breaths every couple of hours.

Observations   How do you feel after a few minutes of massage?

How is your Eye-C vision-fitness? Is it clear at first and then blurry? Can you bring the clarity back?

Combine the eye-muscle stretch with this game. Discover your favorite acupressure points.

What combination of games produces the most exciting results for you?

Phase Three

NOTE: Do not wear a patch when you play the games in this phase.

Phase Three, Activity 15: String Thing

Purpose   To train the brain to accept each eye's perception, and to train the eyes to cooperate in whole-brain perception.

Materials   A ten-foot string and three colored beads. Thread the beads onto the string so that they slide easily along its length.

Instructions   Attach one end of the string to a door handle or other fixture. You can also use a screw-in hook connected to any wooden surface. I have seen string things attached above beds, on verandas, in bathrooms, and in kitchens. The most ingenious setup I have seen is the string tied to a television.

     Pull the string tight and place the free end on the tip of your nose. Make sure that your finger doesn't block the vision of either eye.

     Place one of the wooden beads at the far end next to the knot or point of attachment. Place the next bead halfway down the string, and bring the last bead to your optimum close distance (the point where you

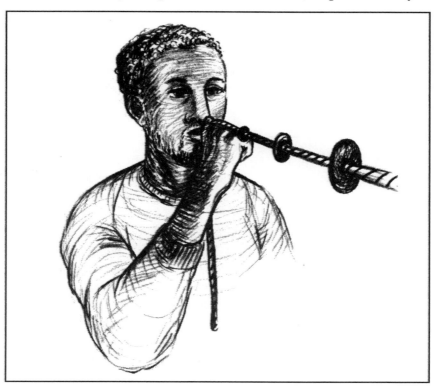

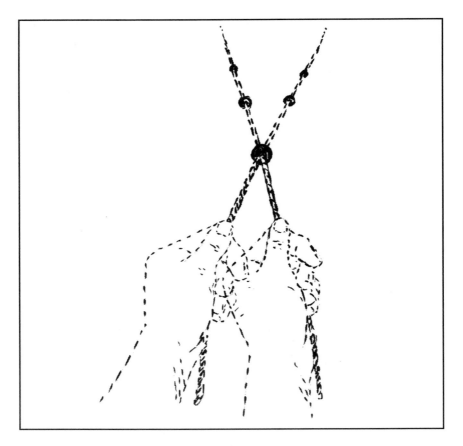

can just make out the detail of the bead; this distance will vary depending on whether you are farsighted or nearsighted). If the close bead becomes unclear, move it away until it clears. Focus your attention (looking) at the closest bead. With both eyes open, and breathing in a relaxed way, get in touch with how your eyes feel while looking at the bead.

Can you see one bead, or does it slip into two images? Do you feel any strain or tension in your eye muscles? While looking at the closest bead, can you see what is going on behind that bead?

The answers to these questions will help you to understand your level of vision-fitness.

If you can balance your looking and seeing, you will notice that the distant beads appear double.

You may also see two strings radiating from the near bead in both directions. This is a good sign. It means that your eyes are working together and that your brain is accepting both images.

If any parts of the string disappear, then parts of visual space are being suppressed. This could mean that your subconscious does not want to see part of what is in your world.

If any of the distant beads disappear, this indicates that the brain cannot simultaneously handle input from both eyes.

Attempt to bring the near bead closer to your nose. If you can maintain an image of one bead, your vision-fitness is good. If the bead begins slipping into two, then play the game more often until you achieve mastery.

String thing is an excellent game to play with preschool children to prepare them to learn to read.

You can use string thing to verify your vision-fitness after working at a computer terminal.

Play the game for twenty to thirty breaths, then zoom to other beads, and finally palm.

Observations
Under what conditions do the beads or parts of the string disappear?

When you incorporate spelling, talking, or thinking, what happens to the string(s) or the beads? When you let your mind wander for a moment, what happens?

Zoom back and forth between the different beads. Maintain one bead where you are "looking" and two beads where you are "seeing."

Close your eyes and imagine the position of the beads. In your mind's eye, zoom back and forth between the beads.

Do you have more stamina after playing the game?

Phase Three, Activity 16: Fencing

Purpose   To extend the concepts learned from Activity 15 into
             space and your daily life. To train your brain and eyes
             to look and see simultaneously.

Materials   A thirty-two-inch piece of flexible, plastic-covered
             electrical wire.

Instructions Following the diagram, bend the wire to custom-fit
             your head. The goal is to have a two-inch-long piece
             of wire hanging about six inches in front of your eyes.
             This wire is called a fence post in this game.

             As in string thing, when you look past the single
             fence post, observe that there now appear to be two.
             Whatever you are looking at, place that object exactly
             between the fence posts.

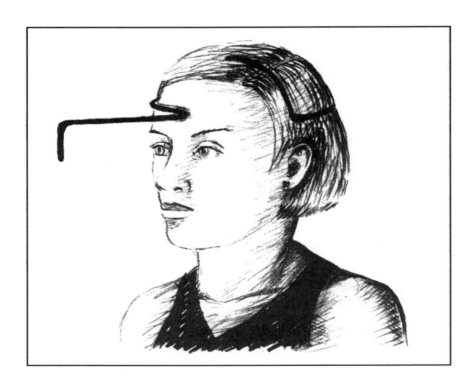

Make sure that both fence posts are present all the time. If not, blink your eyes, take a deep breath, aim your eyes toward the single fence post, and then relax. The second fence post should return. If it doesn't, remove the gadget and palm your eyes, stretch the muscles, massage the face, and yawn. Repeat until you see two fence posts. (NOTE: *If you are unable to elicit two fence posts, your vision-fitness may be too low for you to master fencing at this time. Continue working on earlier games until your vision-fitness increases.*) Walk around the room placing objects between the fence posts. The goal, as before, is to be able to look and see. What you look at appears single, and what you see appears double.

Look out of a window and imagine that you can see across the street, to the other side of the city, outside your state, across the country.

As you imagine looking at a far distance and envision a clear object in that place, notice what happens to the separation of the fence posts.

Visualize that looking farther into space is equivalent to creating more visual space. This is monitored by how far apart you see the fence posts. The farther you look, the greater is the separation between the fence posts. The farther they separate, the more space there is.

As in string thing, imagine that there is a string coming from the object in far space stretching out toward the real (single) fence post.

When you look directly at the fence post, the two posts will merge into one fence post, and your eyes will be crossing. Remember, it is OK to cross your eyes; they will not get stuck, but do not strain them.

There is no time limit to playing fencing.

Observations   How does it feel to look at the fence post and see one?

If you feel any tension or strain, breathe, blink, and palm your eyes for twenty to fifty breaths.

Use the fencing game while you watch television, read, cook, talk with friends, and work at the computer.

Notice under what conditions the two fence posts change. Notice when one fence post fades, becomes blurry, moves, or disappears. Observe whether you want to avoid looking between the two fence posts under certain viewing conditions.

Fencing is a wonderful way to monitor how thinking, distress, and tension affect the way your eyes work together.

Phase Three, Activity 17: Thumb Zapping

See chapter 11 for a description of this game.

Phase Three, Activity 18: Finger Doubling

Purpose   To induce beginning awareness of stereoscopic perception and to further develop whole-brain vision.

Instructions   Place your thumbs one behind the other ten inches in front of your eyes.

While looking far away, perceive two thumbs.

Now place one thumb next to the other thumb and slightly separate them to a distance of about two inches.

Keep looking far away, and notice that you now see either three or four thumbs.

Move your thumbs a little farther apart until you are aware of three thumbs. Keep breathing and blinking to maintain a balanced perception of the three thumbs.

Now zoom your looking to the point where you think there are three thumbs, and you will notice that they go back into two.

Zoom far away and there will once again be three. Practice this zooming until it is easy for you to see three thumbs even while standing on one leg.

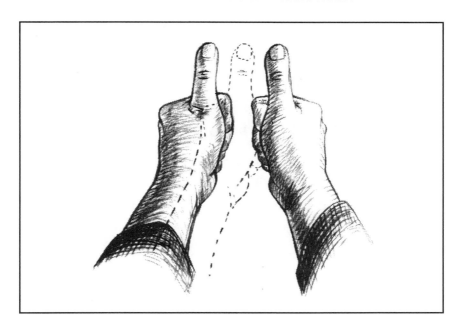

Move your two physical thumbs farther away and then closer, and observe the effect that this has on your ability to maintain three thumbs.

Cross your eyes slightly. By crossing your eyes you will see either three or four thumbs. The goal is to see three and to make the middle thumb as clear as possible.

Place your physical thumbs at different distances from your face and notice how your performance varies.

Next, see if you can look past the physical thumbs and perceive three again. Attempt to zoom behind and in front, getting three thumbs each time.

Spend fifteen minutes, if necessary, to gain mastery.

Observations   Spell different words while zooming to different distances.

Sit in front of the Eye-C chart and notice changes while you zoom and see three thumbs.

Include plenty of palming, pressure points, and yawns.

Phase Three, Activity 19: Circles

See chapter 11 for a description of this game.

Phase Three, Activity 20: Imaging

Purpose To train your inner vision to create pictures of anything you desire.

Instructions Find a quiet place where you can play the imaging game.

Make yourself very relaxed. Enjoy five deep breaths.

Image yourself at your current age. See your home, animals, bedroom, and kitchen. See the colors of the walls and your view from different windows.

Image a trip you took last summer. Experience the pictures in vivid colors. Pretend that you can feel objects which you see.

Hear yourself talking to friends, family members, and colleagues.

Go back to any age and repeat the same game.

How well can you see your parents? Can you see them sharing themselves with you? Do you feel love coming from them? Can you pretend that your parents are loving you now?

Begin to see yourself without your eyeglasses or contacts. What would your experience of seeing without eyeglasses be like? How soon can you imagine that happening?

See yourself as a child without eyeglasses.

Image the period about eighteen months prior to first receiving eyeglasses. How much distress did you experience during this period? Let your mind's eye create any pictures you desire of the past, present, or future.

Observations How easy is it for you to image? Can you let your mind just "free flow"? Can you quiet your conscious mind enough to see pictures?

How well can you write about your imaging experience?

How does the imaging game connect to your goals or purposes?

Phase Three, Activity 21: Maintenance Program

Purpose To review the whole program and to decide how you can incorporate the most effective components into your daily life.

Instructions Read your diary and recall the vision games that were most effective for you. Make a list of the activities you would like to continue. Your maintenance program could include relaxation, an imagery tape, patches, vision games, nutrition, aerobic exercise, affirmations, and recordkeeping.

You may wish to use the Eye-C chart once a week and to use patches for specific activities such as reading, bookkeeping, or computer work.

When during the day could you play your favorite vision games? Within one day, you should complete a master list outlining how you intend to continue your *Seeing Without Glasses* program.

Observations Are you keeping up with your program?

Are you seeking follow-up care from your eye doctor?

When do you intend to obtain your next reduced-power lens prescription?

Do you have a friend who might want to repeat the program with you in the future?

Summary of the Vision Games

	Activity	Game
Phase One (one-eyed patch)	1	Zooming
	2	Palming
	3	Eye-C chart
	4	Soft focus
	5	Painting/yawning
	6	Swing ball
	7	Shifting/scanning
Phase Two (two-eyed patch)	8	Nose pencil
	9	Lighting
	10	Dynamic visual meditation
	11	Eye-muscle stretch
	12	Marching
	13	Acupressure
	14	Shoulder and neck massage
Phase Three (no patch)	15	String thing
	16	Fencing
	17	Thumb zapping
	18	Finger doubling
	19	Circles
	20	Imaging
	21	Maintenance program

Chapter 13

Using Pinholes to Improve Your Vision

Pinholes, a plastic frame made up of many small holes, are one of the numerous tools you can use on your journey to better vision. Instead of lenses before your eyes, you look through lots of little holes. A full aviator style is used for near and farsightedness and a smaller version with slightly larger holes is used for farsightedness after forty. (See Vision-Improvement Programs and Services.)

If you currently wear compensating glasses or contacts, remove them for an interesting experiment. In a safe environment put on the pinholes and notice an improvement in your naked eyesight. In tandem with the vision games described in chapter 12, pinholes will give you an opportunity to rest your eyes by taking breaks from wearing strong eyeglasses or contact lenses.

How the Pinhole Works

The pinhole has been one of the diagnostic tools used by optometrists and ophthalmologists since the early days of eye refraction. As the name implies, the diagnostic pinhole consists of a single hole the size of the head of a pin in the middle of a dark opaque area. When a person with a measurable refractive error of the eye, such as nearsightedness, farsightedness, or astigmatism, looks through the little hole, clearer eyesight can result.

A 1992 press release by the American Academy of Ophthalmology stated, "People with nearsightedness, farsightedness, or astigmatism may temporarily see more clearly while wearing the multiple pinhole glasses."

The pinhole theoretically permits only one ray of light from each point on an object to pass through to the retina of the eye. One might consider that the pinhole is creating an artificially small pupil, thus bypassing normal aberrations and refractive errors of the eye. The resulting increase in eyesight gives the impression of improved vision without conventional eyeglasses or contact lenses. The pinhole allows the doctor to identify blurry vision caused by an error of refraction, against the presence of a diseased condition in the eyes.

In refractive errors like nearsightedness, farsightedness, or astigmatism, the pinhole results in improved vision when no eye disease exists. When an eye disease is present, the pinhole may not allow the person to see sharper images.

Since the pinholes artificially eliminate a significant amount of the refractive error, there is a potential illusion that the pinholes could improve vision if worn all the time. This is not necessarily the case. It depends on how relaxed you are while wearing the pinholes.

Historically, the wearing of glasses was designed to permit the natural function of the eye to begin a healing process, which would later result in less dependency on glasses. Research reveals that the contrary is occurring. In the same earlier press release in 1992, the American Academy of Ophthalmology stated, "Eyes are neither strengthened nor weakened by glasses. Using your eyes will not damage them, whether or not you are wearing your glasses."

It would appear that wearing eyeglasses or contact lenses should correct your vision. Most eyeglass and contact-lens wearers will refute this claim. The more the eyeglasses are worn, the more dependent the eyes become to the external aid that provides the clearness.

Do Pinholes Improve or Correct Vision?

Specifically designed lens prescriptions, combined with a prudently taught vision-fitness program, have in some cases resulted in less dependency on eyeglasses. This is true of some myopia (nearsighted-ness), astigmatism, hyperopia (farsightedness), presbyopia ("old-age" sight), and strabismus (eyes crossing).

Improving vision is dependent on your agreement and commitment to the healing process. Better eyesight does not necessarily mean that there will be immediate significant reductions in the measured nearsightedness, farsightedness, or astigmatism dioptric readings obtained by your optometrist or ophthalmologist. Increases in vision and eyesight capacity occur in the brain and mind and are perceptual in nature. Significant improvements in the brain's perceptions can occur in an eyeball that is diagnosed as farsighted, nearsighted, or astigmatic. Vision-fitness training can permit you to see more clearly.

Vision researchers have called for more attention to the role of the mind and the brain in vision. Structural changes in the eye do not show up as quickly as the functional and perceptual changes in the mind. This is the eyesight part of vision. The lag time between the functional and structural changes may be as long as nine months to three years. I have personally conducted research in this field. Lens prescriptions that are reduced when combined with a rational vision-fitness program, such as the use of pinholes, in conjunction with the following vision games do create statistically significant improvements in eyesight. Reduced dependence on strong eyeglasses does result. This is in spite of no or minimal refractive changes being measurable in the eye.

The eye is an extension of the brain, which functions in harmony with all the other aspects of the central and autonomic nervous systems. The food you eat, your attitude, and the amount of exercise your body receives all can have a bearing on your vision. External aids will not "miraculously" cure your poor eyesight.

If you are a highly committed individual and use your own inner capacity, while combining proven visual aids such as pinholes and vision-fitness lens prescriptions, true improvements in your vision can occur. As part of a responsible vision-fitness program, pinholes can be extremely beneficial by increasing the effectiveness of your eyesight in daily living. When you choose to actively participate in your vision care, actual changes in your eye structure can be measured. The pinholes give a respite from your strong eyeglass prescription and allow you to function with clearer eyesight than is possible with your unassisted eyes. With the implementation of vision-fitness training, naked vision (without lenses or pinholes) can show improvement.

Using the Pinholes in Your Daily Life

When putting on the pinholes, you become aware of how different your perceptions are through them, as compared to the use of eyeglass or contact-lens prescriptions. Your first impression might be one of feeling annoyed or disturbed by the presence of the little holes.

You may find yourself straining or staring through the little holes trying to enjoy the clarity. A tension-like feeling may appear around the brow. Take a series of deep breaths and become aware of how, by consciously breathing, you can relieve any of the tightness or tense feelings in and around the eyes. The basic difference between pinholes and regular contact-lens and eyeglass prescriptions is that you have to participate more when looking through the pinholes. By that, I mean you will find it necessary to adjust the posture of your head and look through and around the little holes.

The training effect of the pinholes is that you have to be more present while using and wearing them. This participation and interaction between you and the pinholes can facilitate the improvement of your vision. As long as you stay aware and look through the holes, the strain or discomfort will be minor and the annoyance of the holes will go away. As this happens, you will experience more "normal" vision while looking through the little holes. (The holes seem to lose their dark borders, and you can see through them easily.) When this happens you are expanding your sense of visual space. Use the pinholes as a relaxation exercise, a time away from your busy schedule, where you can practice "being" more than "doing." Experiment with relaxing your mind and notice how the little holes seem to bother you less. Go for a walk in familiar surroundings.

Breathing and Blinking

Remember to keep blinking and breathing. It is permissible to not blink for ten or fifteen seconds to orient and align your head position until such time that your looking through the pinholes provides clear single vision. Thereafter, begin consciously blinking every three to five seconds as you begin to move your eyes around, scanning different distances both for close and faraway vision.

It is your active participation while looking through the pinholes that facilitates the improvement of your vision. Let your mind become so relaxed that you hardly notice the little holes. It will feel as if you are stretching your vision to go farther away or to focus closer. Be careful if you are walking around with the pinholes, lest you bump into something or trip. In the beginning, wear them only while you are sitting down. Later, experiment walking, watching a movie, or even working at a computer.

Precautions

Wear the pinholes only in non-life-threatening situations. Do not use them while driving, working around mechanical or electrical devices, when using knives or instruments, or when you are tired. If you have any questions about the health of your eyes or compensating lens prescriptions, please consult with your optometrist or ophthalmologist.

When first putting on the pinholes, please be aware that there is an adjustment period. The brain needs to adjust to the new perceptions. Begin with short periods of five to twenty minutes only. When you take them off, notice the increase in your eyes' light sensitivity and perception.

While you are wearing the pinholes, note that your eyes are beginning to relax behind the holes as you breathe and blink. Spend a few moments fine-tuning your breathing and blinking every three to five seconds. Keep both eyes open even though there may be a tendency to feel that one eye is "the preferred eye," or the dominating one.

There is a small probability that if you are not consciously aware of your breathing and blinking exercises, your perception through both eyes may not be integrated. The movement of the eyes, coupled with the breathing and blinking, provides a high degree of integration, at the level of the brain, from the light and messages traveling through the eyes. Become aware of any straining, tiredness, or tension that may build up in your eyes.

Nearsightedness, Farsightedness, Astigmatism, and Other Diagnosed Eye Conditions

Depending on the eye condition diagnosed by your optometrist or ophthalmologist, the way you use the pinholes may vary.

Nearsightedness (Myopia)

If you are nearsighted, the pinholes can be worn primarily when looking into the far distance. The aim is to look far away and beyond the holes while maintaining a relaxed perception. The farther you can train yourself to look into the distance, the more effective the vision benefits will be after you remove the pinholes. Unless you also have farsightedness (hyperopia) and you are over the age of forty-five, you would probably spend more time looking far away through the pinholes than looking close-up for reading.

Experiment now by looking at some written material with small print, with your naked vision and with the pinholes, to determine your need for using them for close reading. If the pinholes increase the clarity of small print, then use them also for close work.

"Old-Age" Sight or "Short-Arm" Syndrome

If you have these conditions, or have been diagnosed with them, you will use the "half eye" pinholes (which are smaller so you can look over the top for far viewing) primarily for looking at objects that are close by, such as written materials, books, or computers. Place the reading material approximately sixteen inches from your eyes and adjust your head position until you find one central spot where, with both eyes open, the written material appears to be clear and sharply in focus. Increase the room lighting, if necessary. And remember to breathe and blink.

As you take a few connected breaths, you may be aware of how the small print pops into focus more quickly after you inhale. The small pinholes permit a centering effect on the eyes as well as a clearer focus. Observe how the blackness of the print increases and how you can see even the grain of the paper. As you wear the pinholes, imagine that your naked vision without lenses or pinholes can be just as clear. Explore the physical and emotional variables that are present when your vision is this clear versus when your vision appears more blurry. This procedure will give you great insight about how your mind affects your clear vision.

Astigmatism

In this particular condition, the curvature of the cornea is different in one direction compared to another. This could be producing varying degrees of visual blurriness in your eyesight. Astigmatism results in a greater distortion or blurriness in one orientation of your gaze (vertical or horizontal). Usually, the distorted shape of the outside eye structure of the cornea reflects this astigmatism. The pinholes bypass the corneal distortion and resulting blurriness, and a clear focus in all orientations of gaze is maintained. While looking at small print or looking off into the distance, move your eyes in a horizontal direction, a vertical direction, and then a diagonal direction while you breathe and blink.

Do you feel that one of these eye movements feels more uncomfortable than another? Practice the one that feels the most difficult. More than likely, the meridian that feels the most uncomfortable or jerky is the most blurry orientation of your vision. As you practice moving your eyes along this meridian, you will be activating your inner vision, which is a form of self-healing. That specific eye movement is like a homeopathic remedy that activates the eye muscles, which, in turn, stimulate the nerves from the brain and then focuses your attention on the part of your mind where 90 percent of vision happens.

Diagnosed Eye Conditions

In some cases of diagnosed cataracts, glaucoma, macular degeneration, retinal detachments, retinitis pigmentosa, and other debilitating eye conditions, the pinholes may prove beneficial in sharpening your eyesight. Slip on the pinholes and become aware, while reading fine print or looking farther away, whether objects appear sharper and clearer. If this does happen, there is a high probability that, irrespective of the eye condition, you have functional vision that can be helped by using the pinholes, specially designed lens prescriptions, and/or vision-fitness games or exercises. The pinholes will then prove to be a useful adjunct to other treatments that are being provided by your eye doctor or that you are gleaning from our materials, tapes, and books. If not, please consider the recommendations in chapter 14.

Freeing Yourself from Strong Eyeglasses or Contact Lenses

If your desire is to improve your vision and be less dependent on eyeglass prescriptions, the pinholes will permit you to spend less time wearing the strong lens prescriptions. The advantage of this is that wearing the pinholes breaks up the habitual state of the brain that was becoming accustomed to strong compensating lenses. Also, pinholes ease the transition to the full blur of the naked vision state, which most people find difficult to deal with.

Many pinhole users have found that supplementing the natural light entering the eyes with full-spectrum fluorescent tubes or color-corrected balanced incandescent light bulbs is useful support for maintaining the increased sharpness present with pinholes. Remember, it is important to use good lighting while using the pinholes because there is a restriction and diminishing of the natural light present. Also, when removing the pinholes, spend time monitoring the improvements in your vision-fitness by using an eyechart like the Eye-C charts (see Vision-Improvement Programs and Services). It is apparent that the percentage increase in clarity while looking through the pinholes is between 45 percent and 60 percent. The real benefit would be to maintain this clarity after removing the pinholes. The activities which follow will ensure that you can continue increasing your eyesight after removing the pinholes.

Zooming and Palming

While looking through the pinholes, focus your eyes on the little holes and then on an object far beyond the holes. This vision game is called zooming. These practices are a review of what you have learned in chapter 12 but specifically for use with the pinholes. If this does not alleviate the strain, remove the pinholes, rub your palms together, and place them over your closed eyelids. Breathing for approximately ten to twenty breaths and gently keeping your palms over your eyes should alleviate any tension or strained feeling in the eyes. Then put the pinholes on once again. After looking through the pinholes for a while outdoors, close your eyes and become aware of the alternating dark and light lines or after-images in front of your eyes that will be seen through your closed eyelids.

This after-image effect is a demonstration of how the light coming through the little holes stimulates a particular part of the retina, while parts of the dark area (the black plastic) prevent light from coming in. The alternation between light coming in and light being blocked creates this after-image. This retinal effect, an additional vision-improvement stimulation, can increase the conversion of the light energy into photoelectric neural impulses. As you can see, many aspects of awareness can be used to keep you consciously participating in the act of improving your vision while wearing the pinholes.

Covering of One Eye

Should you become aware that there is a major difference between the left-eye perception and the right-eye perception, you may wish to place some masking tape or sticky translucent tape on the inside of the pinholes over the eye that is the "stronger." This will create an opportunity for you to train your vision through the "weaker" eye.

Zooming can be extremely beneficial for enhancing the perception through the less-clear eye to increase the vision-fitness to the point where it more closely matches that of the clearer perceiving eye (at least no more than 15 percent difference). While looking through one eye and focusing your eyes on the little holes, you will notice that the blackness of the surrounding area of the hole appears much darker when you are focused on the little hole. When you then release your focus and look toward the far-distant object, you will notice less of a dark area around the little hole, as if there is more white light present to enable you to see farther away. The object of the game is to zoom your focus to the little hole and then zoom it away, back and forth, as you breathe to stimulate the focusing ciliary muscle as well as the lens and the fovea of your eye.

Repeat this for ten to twenty breaths, then take off the pinholes and palm your eyes as before for an additional ten to twenty breaths. During this zooming game, the little holes will appear to pulsate back and forth as the focus of your eye changes. It is this focusing mechanism (ciliary muscle) that becomes sluggish and "out of shape." By using the pinholes to monitor the positive aspect of zooming your focus, you will be directly affecting the vision-fitness of your focusing muscle. The muscle in the iris of your eye will also be stimulated, and specific neural energy will be sent to the fovea of that eye. Once you have noticed more balance in the way the left and right eyes see individually (check your progress on the Distance or Near Eye-C chart by covering one eye and then the other and comparing the difference), repeat the vision game without the tape, with both eyes open. You will notice that it may be more difficult to zoom your focus with both eyes open than with just using one eye. The reason is that when you focus with both eyes open, there is also a tendency to cross the eyes. This game will be explained in more detail below under "Eye Crossing."

Eye-Muscle Stretch

While wearing the pinholes and breathing, move your eyes in a horizontal direction, as far to the right and then left as possible without straining, following the little holes as you move from left to right. (*NOTE: If you are very nearsighted, five diopters or more, be very careful not to stretch your eyes too far as it may lead to detaching the retina.*)

Repeat this for approximately five breaths, then do it in the vertical direction, letting the eyes follow the holes up and down. Repeat for the diagonal motions for five breaths up to the left and down to the right and then up into the right and down into the left.

After completion of each sequence of five breaths, allow the eyes to zoom far away through the little holes into the distance or at some reading material close by. You will feel that the motion of the eyes creates a form of relaxation and flexibility that is helpful in improving your vision. After you have completed the sequence, allow your eyes to make a very large circle around the pinholes, always being aware of the pinholes while you are moving in a clockwise and then counter-clockwise direction, approximately five breaths each way.

After a strenuous fitness technique like this, take the pinholes off and palm your eyes for ten to twenty breaths. Before placing the pinholes back in front of your eyes, allow the fingers of each hand to press along the eyebrow margin, moving from the inside toward the outside. This action is stimulating acupressure points along the meridian of the eyebrow. Repeat this for five to ten breaths.

Thumb Zapping

While looking through the pinholes at a point far away, choose a particular object that stands out from the rest of the environment. Place your thumb between your eyes and the object you are looking at. While blinking and breathing and maintaining a fixed focus on the distant object, become aware that there are probably two thumbs visible. If this is not the case, keep blinking and breathing in an attempt to make yourself see two thumbs while looking far past the thumbs. If you cannot accomplish this, it might mean your eyes are not sending equal messages to the brain and, therefore, your brain is not able to create two-eyed perception. You will not be able to advance to the next phase of the vision game until your two eyes are more able to cooperate. Continue covering the eye with the "less clear" vision. Assuming that you are aware of two thumbs, notice if one thumb is higher than the other. Adjust your head by cocking your earlobe toward the right shoulder or the left shoulder until the two thumbs appear equally high. Maintain a breathing and blinking pattern that visibly sustains the presence of the two thumbs. Practice looking beyond the holes, attempting to gauge yourself looking toward points farther away from you. The farther away you can look, the less apparent the holes will be.

Thumb Zooming

After you have mastered this phase, change your point of looking and focus on your extended thumb. You will notice that the two thumbs now come into one image and the object beyond the thumb now appears to be two images. Repeat this zooming from your thumb to the object, back and forth, always maintaining the awareness of there being two images where you are not looking directly. While zooming and practicing the thumb-zapping awareness, watch the appearance of the little holes. While you are looking at the thumb, the borders of the hole will appear more filled in and darker. When you then zoom out, it appears that you are seeing through the holes, such that it seems you have more space in the holes to look through. Repeat this vision game until you can maintain the awareness of the increased darkness while looking at the thumb and the image of the lesser darkness while looking far away.

Eye Crossing

When you have mastered the techniques up to this point, attempt to see the object far away as two without the presence of the thumb at all. That is, align your gaze where the thumb used to be and maintain the appearance of double vision far away. (*NOTE: There is no danger of your eyes becoming stuck while you do the eye-crossing vision game, even though you may have been told that as a child.*)

You can maintain the appearance of double vision by tuning in to the darkness of the circles as you adjust your focus to the place where the thumb used to be. As you adjust your eye-crossing closer and closer to the little holes, the distance of the double object widens while the little holes begin to overlap each other.

By practicing the eye-crossing and thumb-zapping game, you are training your eye-muscle flexibility, which helps the eyes cross inward as well as sharpening the precision of the focus of the ciliary muscle. Stimulating the outside and inside muscles is most desirable for the eyes to work together as a team. Do this for ten breaths. Notice that while crossing your eyes, everything far away also seems to become smaller.

After you have completed this exercise, remove the pinholes and check your vision-fitness looking through a window, calendar, painting, or the Distance or Near Eye-C chart, far away and up close without pinholes. It is quite common and most gratifying for an increase in vision-fitness to occur as a result of this vision game.

Advanced Eye Crossing

Choose an object far away and, with the pinholes in place, align that object through the center of one of the little holes in the central portion of your line of vision. Cross your eyes a little and observe that the object now has a double counterpart within its own little hole off to the side. By crossing the eyes even more, notice that eventually a third hole and finally a fourth hole appear. Also, whatever you can see through the subsequent little holes will be brilliantly sharp, as if you were seeing through a telescope. Repeat this vision game with the breathing and blinking techniques while looking at different objects. Zoom back and forth to one object, and then blink and go to another object. To avoid stinging, burning, and eyestrain symptoms, include lots of palming, breathing, and blinking during this vision game. You can also stimulate the pressure points with your fingers.

If You Use a Computer

Let the computer screen act as the thumb or point of eye crossing while placing a Distance Eye-C chart on the wall behind the screen. After each fifty-five-minute period of looking at the screen, take a five-minute break and practice the vision games, or take one minute off each twenty minutes.

Daily Use of the Pinholes and Vision-Fitness

Attempt to spend at least fifteen minutes each day using the pinholes and incorporating the vision games into your daily living. Use the pinholes while you walk, watch television, garden, read, and in the other daily activities that do not require your full attention. Begin with short periods (fifteen minutes) and extend by five-minute intervals. Do not spend more than thirty to sixty minutes at a time wearing the pinholes without taking palming or zooming breaks. Remember that you cannot damage your eyes by exercising them while being conscious and aware of how you use them and when you feel eyestrain.

Summary of Vision Games While Wearing Pinholes

It is best to use breaths as a way to time yourself in the varying phases of improving your vision.

- Decide when you can wear your pinholes instead of your strong eyeglasses. Begin with ten-minute periods in non-life-threatening situations and build up to sixty minutes.

- Put pinholes on. Breathe and blink. Take fifteen to thirty breaths.

- Use a Distance or Near Eye-C chart to monitor improvements in vision.

- Practice looking beyond the holes, either at near or far distances, for twenty breaths.

- If you have been told that you have astigmatism, move your eyes in different horizontal, vertical, or diagonal directions.

- Zoom your vision for ten breaths.

- Palm your eyes for twenty breaths.

- If necessary, cover one eye for up to one hour.

- Begin to understand the anatomy of your eyes.

Advanced Vision Games

- Eye-muscle stretch—thirty breaths

- Thumb zapping—twenty breaths

- Eye crossing—twenty breaths

- Thumb zooming—twenty breaths

Chapter 14

Help for Eye-Disease Conditions

"There is nothing you can do to help this eye condition!" These self-defeating words have echoed the walls of many eye doctors' offices all over the world. Is it true what most doctors say? No! Some useful visual function can usually be regained no matter what the diagnosis has been. I always encourage individuals to seek a second opinion.

The basic question is this: "Are there ways to restore natural eye function in the presence of a disease?" My answer is yes.

My opinion and recommendations are based on many years of practical observation and interaction with clients. Hearing negative and "no hope" opinions can affect your body's ability to conduct its own natural healing, especially when "bad news" is being conveyed.

Hearing that there is something you can do to help yourself is enough to awaken your ability to continue your own healing. In my practice, the connection between the patient and me is quite healing in itself. By opening my heart and sharing, I create a safe environment for my clients to shift their perspectives of their eye conditions. I wish this for you as well.

Can people actually restore natural eye function in the presence of a disease? Yes. I have seen it occur. The actual measurable results from natural therapies for improving eye conditions are mixed because few individuals are dedicated enough to earnestly follow the program. My initial approach with my clients is not to just give them "things" to do. I ask them to look at their eye condition as a special messenger to wake them up to their subconscious mind. In other words, the eye disease condition is actually reflecting what is going on in your life and is asking you to look seriously into your lifestyle, attitudes, and beliefs.

You can begin by changing your point of view about your eye condition. Understand that it has occurred in response to some subconscious beliefs about your life. Are you denying some important inner feelings or needs in your life? I am sure you have heard about people who lead very busy and productive lives, and suddenly they have an accident or they fall ill. Their lives quickly grind to a complete halt and they have no choice but to slow down and take stock of themselves and their life direction. An eye-disease condition is a perfect opportunity to take a close look at yourself and how you live your life and make any appropriate changes.

What Are Your Eyes Telling You?

What message is your eye condition attempting to communicate to you? If you were to change your life, what would you do differently? Take a close look at your life as it is today. Don't wait for your eye condition to be so advanced that you are forced to make changes in your life.

Many of my new clients express their fear of going blind. It is not so much that they fear the blindness but how their lives are going to change. They express concerns of not being able to drive, read, or watch television. In the case of macular degeneration, where a person has difficulty reading because of a central blind area, could the message be for him to stop reading? What would he do with his life if he were not reading? The person would have to face himself, and the fears, incompletions, and all the unconsciousness in his personal life. Would it be helpful for those with glaucoma to begin looking at the areas in their life where they put themselves under too much pressure?

When you begin to look at eye disease as a positive experience, it awakens you to all the blindness you create in your life. You have the choice to wake up and change direction. The eye disease is like an alarm system that is warning you to please begin seeing what your life is really about with clarity and focus.

Where Do I Begin?

There is more to life than what the majority of the world seems to accept. In order to deal with the reality of your eye disease you can combine your choices. First, you can consult your conventional eye doctor, who will offer you external medications or surgery. The doctor may have said that nothing can be done. Start being responsible for your own visual well-being. In addition to your doctor's suggestions, you can empower yourself to begin looking deeply inside and find your own solutions. Go beyond what you think is true for you. Go into the truth of the feelings in your own heart, and stay out of your intellectual and rational mind for a while. The answers lie inside of you, and not only in your thinking. Begin sharing honestly about your feelings and the clarity you wish to bring into your life.

These suggestions open the door for a wonderful experience— the preliminary inner work you undertake by going into the root of your feelings and needs is the preparation for the practical application. Begin by exploring the reasons you have experienced blurriness or blindness in the past, reasons that may be contributing to your eye disease. Some examples are suppressed emotional hurt, relocating, divorce, separation, changing jobs, death of a friend or spouse, retirement, demotion, cut in salary, and illness. What was going on in your life at about the time your condition was first diagnosed, or when you experienced the first symptoms? By undertaking this journey you open up to the possibility of creating positive changes in your eye condition.

Relationship to Life and Death

Another important aspect of eye disease that I constantly come across in my practice is how my clients relate to life and their ultimate death. In the older days, eye-disease conditions were present mostly in the elderly; however, things have changed, and nowadays I see many young people with the same eye diagnoses.

Seniors who are approaching the completion of life in their physical body tell me about their fears of dying. I wonder if their eye conditions, metaphorically speaking, represents a form of blindness. Eye disease forces people to slow down and pay attention to their real purpose for living. If you are busy with the material things in life, perhaps your eye condition is offering you the ideal opportunity to explore the spiritual side of living and dying, which may be as helpful to you as it has been to many of my clients.

If your eye condition progressed to its full maturity and you became blind, what would your life be like then? How would you modify your lifestyle and open yourself to other ways of being in life? In this worst-case scenario, living with an eye disease or going blind doesn't have to be a nightmare. It could be a very liberating experience. Many people who have had to endure harsh adversity in the years before they became blind have turned their lives around and achieved great success. Perhaps your eye condition is your chance to reevaluate your life's direction and purpose. Even if you never improve your eye condition, there may be some incredible value to be gained from your hardship. Perhaps this is the time to reclaim a lost dream or aspiration.

My approach to dealing with life-debilitating eye conditions goes beyond the approach of trying to find a remedy or "fix-it-up," which is so common in our modern culture. You can't say, "I'll just put in a new eye part or have the old eye reconditioned with a laser beam!" and not deal with the reason you have the eye disease in the first place. You need to look at your eye disease as a communication from an inner part of yourself that you must address. The external tools do have value; however, they will only be effective if you also do the inner work I am suggesting. Quite often, a surgical intervention offers hope and good results, which may suffice for a while and then, wham, another disease condition surfaces because the person has not dealt with the core issues facing him or her. If you are one of the fortunate people who can turn your eye condition around and regain functional vision, will your vision through your eyes lead you into a new life?

Integrated Vision-Fitness Training

The types of eye conditions that do respond to what I call vision-fitness training are macular degeneration, glaucoma, cataracts, and conditions of the retina, lens, cornea, sclera, iris, optic nerve, and muscles. Please note that the aim of this training is not to treat the physical condition of your eye but to awaken your self-healing ability and encourage a healthy attitude about what is possible beyond the conventional approaches of medical science. This approach is complementary, utilizing educational tools and combining as many as twenty-five different health principles. The preventive and rehabilitative tools are in no way meant to replace conventional medicine. Rather, you are encouraged to use these training tools as an adjunct to your conventional form of vision care. I invite you to become an active participant in your vision-care program and make a commitment to helping yourself improve your vision and eye health.

Spend a moment reconsidering your eye condition. Go back in time to when you first experienced eye symptoms. Recall what was going on in your life twelve to eighteen months prior to those symptoms. Attempt to isolate specific events that were both trying and challenging.

Now, think back to when you were in your eye doctor's office. How did you feel about his diagnosis? Was he or she supportive or perhaps a little distant and cold in the way he or she communicated the "bad news"? Did you feel the doctor understood how you felt when you heard you could potentially become blind or did you feel he was just doing his job? To come to a better understanding about why you even have an eye-disease condition, these observations are important. If you feel any emotion or incompletion with the eye doctor, release those feelings now, as the doctor probably did the best that he or she could at that time. Clinical research is showing that your doctor's support, or lack of it, can strongly influence your perceptions and ability to heal your condition.

Become informed about complementary methods for helping your eye condition. What follows are three primary ways of enhancing your visual wellness based on the complementary approach.

1. Start eating healthy foods, rich in nutrients, that will supply your blood with therapeutic levels of vitamins and minerals. Your blood will, in turn, nourish your eye parts. In addition, you will likely need therapeutic supplements during this process.

2. You may use colored gel filters in goggles and sunlight or a light source directed into your eyes, which become healing tools to mobilize your own self-healing. (See Vision-Improvement Programs and Services. Use the Color Balancing Kit in conjunction with self-healing audiotapes.)

Light and color stimulate the flow of blood and encourage damaged tissue to achieve greater degrees of functionality. The relaxing effect of colored light can, for example, assist you to learn how to lower the pressure inside your eyes, such as is experienced with glaucoma. You can also begin creating a new relationship with sunlight. This amazing energy force provides the food for plants to grow and living things to sustain themselves. In spite of the myopic viewpoint of most health authorities who vehemently claim that sunlight will hurt you, there is ample evidence stating the exact opposite. Some claim that without any sunlight, you will not only become blind, you will die. Sunlight vitalizes your eyes and your general well-being. Your eyes are one of the primary entry points for light and color to reach your nervous system. Your autonomic nervous system regulates all the major balance points within your body and eyes.

3. Bearing in mind that 90 percent of what we perceive comes from the mind and only 10 percent is from the eyes, you can reprogram your mind to see clearly. Your life experiences are likened to computer software that is stored in your brain, and you may be functioning with software that is outdated or no longer useful. Yes, it did serve you some time ago, but do you still need to live by the old programming? The self-healing and personalized audiotapes are the keys to accomplish this. (See Vision-Improvement Programs and Services. Specify your eye condition so the correct tape can be sent to you.)

It is not uncommon for my clients with diagnosed eye-disease conditions to discover that past-stored experiences do affect their current way of looking at life. The eye seems to print out those misperceptions in the form of eye conditions, and in the less severe cases, it can be relatively harmless—a little blurry vision or discomfort around the eye area. My research tells me that when you don't pay attention to the early printouts, the messages begin to intensify. I consider an eye disease to be an amplified alert signal from your inner mind. The initial condition, like nearsightedness, may be a simplified version of the signal. Through the eye disease, the message is printing out loud and clear. Are you willing to pay attention and explore the meaning of the condition and what it is attempting to tell you, or are you going to be like the majority of people and believe that there is nothing you can do to help your two eyes?

Your choices are clear. Pay attention to what your eyes are trying to tell you, or continue covering up the urgent message by wearing glasses, taking eye medication, or undergoing eye surgery. You cannot deny the wondrous nature of your eyes and body. You can break a bone, cut yourself, pull a tendon, hurt a muscle, and your body regenerates. Why should your eyes be any different?

If you apply the principles outlined above, there is no medical reason why your eye function cannot improve. It is a matter of your making the decision to believe and then applying the new information. With patience, you will begin to live the new habits and learn how to look with "new" eyes at your world, defining the new vision of the way you intend to live.

Step-by-Step Suggestions for Seeing Without Glasses

To begin your program of vision improvement, follow these step-by-step suggestions. Take as long as you need before moving on to the next phase. You do not necessarily need to follow the steps in order. Feel free to jump around if a particular phase catches your attention.

- Read the first three parts of this book.

- Make notes of realizations, awarenesses, and ideas in your journal.

- If you wear contact lenses and have backup glasses, begin wearing your glasses.

- If you don't own extra eyeglasses, obtain a transitional pair that will compensate your vision to 20/25.

- If you wear eyeglasses, ask an empathetic eye doctor to prescribe 20/40 vision-fitness lenses for you.

- Determine your vision-fitness from the questionnaire in chapter 1.

- Obtain baseline vision-fitness measurements from chapter 1 and the Eye-C charts on pages 107 and 108.

- Determine your visual style from the exercise in chapter 5.

- Consider modifying your nutritional intake according to the suggestions in chapter 6.

- Consider incorporating aerobic activities into your schedule.

- Systematically increase the amount of time you spend per day without your contacts or glasses. Note which activities you can successfully undertake without wearing eyeglasses or contacts.

- Play the vision games in chapter 11 in order to further assist you in understanding your vision-fitness.

- Spend about a week preparing your personal purposes and goals.

- Spend ten to twenty minutes per day for about a week playing the Eye-C chart game, incorporating the affirmations on pages 90 and 91.

- Spend fifteen minutes per day for about a week outside in natural light without eyeglasses, playing the Activity 9 vision game.

- Begin to wear the one-eyed patch over your preferred (dominant) eye. Determine how long you can comfortably wear the patch by covering the vision-fitness eyeglass lens of your preferred eye or by not using eyeglasses and wearing a patch with a humorous decal or sticker on it as a reminder for you and others that this is a fun-and-games activity rather than an indication that something is wrong with your eye. Try to wear the patch for four hours at a time, but reduce the wearing time if you experience discomfort, and build up to the optimal wearing time by increasing the amount of time you wear the patch each day. (*NOTE: Do not wear the patch under life-threatening conditions such as driving. Begin by wearing the patch in the safety of your home, and when you feel comfortable you can experiment.*)

- Begin the Phase One vision games without your lenses in order to familiarize yourself with the content and directions for the one-eyed vision games. Reread the instructions for the seven vision games in this phase until you are familiar with the content. When you have internalized the information, you can begin to incorporate these vision games into your daily life.

- Repeat the process for the vision games in Phase Two and Phase Three. When you are familiar with all the vision games, practice your favorite games on a daily basis for fifteen minutes.

- Keep vision records as outlined in chapter 12.

- Revisit your eye doctor if necessary.

- If you have questions, I can assist you via a phone consultation.

Epilogue: World's-Eye View

Our home, planet Earth, is going through a major cleansing, and those of us who are ready to see it are being called to face the problems of blindness and denial that are all around us. There is an ever-increasing need for us to see clearly—without the distortion of our glasses or our mental judgments. Unnecessary killing, chopping down precious forests, and contaminating the Earth's soil with chemical waste are some examples of our blindness. We are paying for our past unconsciousness both externally and internally. Our health and vitality are suffering. Vision problems, disease, and nearsightedness are rampant among both young and old. The effects of television, childhood abuse, dysfunctional families, insufficient nurturing, and other modern-day problems are revealing themselves in the breakdown of our eyes and an inability to convey vision as we once could.

It is my sincerest hope that this book will provide the tools necessary to restore visual sensitivity to those who are ready to have a clear outlook. I know that you will share this with others, and in that way the planet will become a better place. If you are in touch with people in politically powerful places, please share this book with them. We need our politicians and healthcare providers to see the process of leadership clearly and to change. Thank you for reading and implementing this knowledge.

Wherever you look, see love and peace!

Roberto Kaplan

Appendix

The clinical research discussed below was conducted at Pacific University's Portland Optometric Clinic during the fall of 1982. These research findings were reported in a paper presented at the 1982 Annual Meeting of the American Academy of Optometry in Chicago. Dr. Brian Henson collaborated in the compilation of the statistical findings.

Subject Selection

Subjects for the clinical investigation were chosen by random selection from respondents to a newspaper advertisement and word of mouth. Potential subjects were screened by optometric examination to find current levels of refractive error, muscle balance, stereopsis, and amounts of presbyopia, if any. (Only myopic and presbyopic subjects were chosen for the study.)

Subjects were given written and verbal information about the purpose of the study, the time involved, and the commitments they needed to make. The optometric measurements were made by optometric interns supervised by clinical optometrists. At the time of the testing, neither the interns nor the subjects knew whether candidates were part of an experimental or control group.

The investigator randomly chose participants for the experimental group and brought them together for a weekend orientation. At that point they were informed that they were the experimental group. The orientation included explanations of the human visual system, the difference between sight and vision, use of affirmations, nutrition, aerobic and movement exercise, self-relaxation audiotapes, use of Eye-C charts, and home vision games. Each subject was given a manual that contained much of the material in *Seeing Without Glasses* and all the vision games presented in the format of the three-phase program as well as guidelines for maintaining a commitment to the program.

The subjects were given forms on which to record their daily food consumption, exercise schedules, and Eye-C chart results. The subjects filled out the vision-fitness questionnaire and the visual-style ratings as presented in chapters 1 and 5 of this book.

Subjects were then divided into teams with designated team leaders. These teams acted as support groups throughout the program. Any subject could call a team leader at any time to report problems or concerns. The teams met once a week to report challenges and any other insights or experiences to the team leader, who then called the investigator. In this way there was constant communication between the subjects and the researcher. Any major problems or misunderstandings were dealt with immediately.

The Program

The three-phase program was divided into three one-week periods. The first week was devoted to monocular vision. Subjects wore a patch over one eye for up to four hours per day during their daily routine as long as they felt they were in a safe environment. They played the vision games daily, adding a new game each day. In addition to the games, they were taught breathing and relaxation techniques.

In the second week, the subjects were introduced to two-eyed viewing. Individual custom-made bi-nasal (two-eyed) patches were provided and worn during the games. New games were added to the first week's program. All the games were performed without instrumentation and were easily understood.

The third week was devoted entirely to two-eyed vision. One binocular game was added each day to the previous two weeks' games.

During the three-week period, the subjects kept track of their food intake, aerobic exercise, Eye-C measurements, daily goals, and personal experiences. At the completion of the three weeks, the subjects turned in all their records and set up appointments for the post-testing.

Results

For the post-testing, the experimental and control-group subjects came in for testing at the same time. Optometric interns again undertook the testing without knowing which group the subject was in. Table I shows the breakdown of the control and experimental groups in terms of age, education level, and numbers (n) of myopic and presbyopic subjects.

Table I Subject Data		
	Control	Experimental
Numbers (n)	21	62
Age (mean)	37	34.7
Min. age	25	14
Max. age	64	60
Educational level		
<H.S.		1.7%
H.S.		11.7%
>H.S.		25.0%
B.A., B.S.		41.6%
>B.S.		6.7%
M.A., M.S.		6.7%
>M.S.		6.7%
Myopes	15	50
Presbyopes	6	12

Table II shows the clinical data of the control and experimental groups. The stereopsis and fixation disparity measurements were made with the American Optical Vectograph Slide, polaroid filters, and loose prisms at far and near.

	Control				Experimental			
Test	n	X̄b	X̄a	t	n	X̄b	X̄a	t
Table II **Data of Experimental Group and Control Group**								
V.A. @ far unaided	17	20/75	20/66	.88	44	20/105	20/77	3.877*
Stereopsis through habitual Rx	18	138"	126"	-.638	48	206"	156"	3.15*
Range of prism diopters to fixation disparity @ far	18	4.58	4.52	.09	45	5.2	7.48	-5.38*
Range of prism diopters to fixation disparity @ near	18	6.82	8.65	-1.55	45	27.58	9.02	-2.76*
Vision-fitness score	20	7.55	8.85	-1.37	58	5.82	9.67	-7.17*
% wearing time of 20/20 Rx#					40	78.9%	19.2%	11.66*

X̄b = pre-test score
X̄a = post-test score
* = significant level of at least .05 using two-tailed test and five planned tests
# = unplanned test

The results showed that for the experimental group, visual acuity at far, stereopsis at far, and range of prism diopters around the fixation disparity at far and near all changed for the better between pre- and post-testing. All other optometric data for either group did not change for the better between the two testings.

The vision-fitness score derived from the questionnaire also changed quite significantly for the experimental group. The subjects were asked to record the wearing time of their current eyeglasses during the program. It was found that the percentage wearing time dropped from 78.9 percent to 19.2 percent—a significant drop in eyeglass dependency.

Table III shows the breakdown of the myopic group and the presbyopic group. This shows that the presbyopes as a group did not show any significant changes. They had the same tendencies for improvement as did the group as a whole, but not at an experimentally significant level. Perhaps a larger sample size would reflect these trends.

Table III							
Experimental Group Data for Myopes and Presbyopes							
	Myopes				Presbyopes		
Test	n	X̄b	X̄a	t	n	X̄b	X̄a	t
V.A. @ near unaided	36	20/210	20/77	3.12*	11	20/68	20/61	2.5
V.A. @ near unaided	36	20/26	20/27	.988	8	20/35	20/34	-.32
Stereopsis through habitual Rx	40	194"	150"	2.51	8	240"	187.5"	-1.87
Range of prism diopters to fixation disparity @ far	39	5.1	7.5	-5.18*	6	6	7.7	-1.41
Range of prism diopters to fixation disparity @ near	37	7.82	9.12	2.44	8	6.5	8.56	-1.3
Vision-fitness score	40	5.87	9.98	-7.95*	12	7.75	9.17	-2.05

X̄b = mean pre-test score
X̄a = mean post-test score
* = significant level of at least .05 using two-tailed test and five planned tests

Table IV lists the behaviors that changed significantly and the percentage change from pre- to post-testing from a behavioral questionnaire given to the subjects. They were rated on a scale of 1 to 10, with 1 being a behavior they never noticed and 10 being something they did constantly. Each of the listed behaviors was given at least a 5 on the rating scale.

Table IV Behaviors			
	Number of subjects reporting behavior*		
Behavior	Pre-testing	Post-testing	% change
Skip word or sentences	22	13	41
Reread lines or phrases	30	14	53
Read too slowly	22	13	41
Comprehension poorer as reading is continued or loses interest quickly	15	7	53
Headaches in forehead or temples	14	7	50
Frowns, scowls, or squints	20	14	30
Rest head on arm when writing	5	11	55
Write crookedly and/or poorly spaced	12	7	42

*See text for explanation of rating scale.

Summary

The *Seeing Without Glasses* three-phase program demonstrated that when subjects were supported in applying an interdisciplinary approach to developing vision, they could produce significant changes in their perception as measured by binocular optometric measurements.

While the refractive data did not change significantly, the positive increase in ranges around the fixation disparity can be interpreted as greater tolerance for handling visual stress. This seemed to be confirmed by the behavioral comments from the research subjects.

Behaviors related to general vision skills and fitness of the visual-processing system improved by the time of post-testing. These findings suggest that the visual performance of eye movements, focusing, and binocularity can change in a short home-based vision-training program such as the *Seeing Without Glasses* program.

Conclusions

Since so many variables—nutrition, relaxation, patches, exercise, vision games, support, affirmations, and others—together produced the significant changes, future studies should determine which of the variables effect the changes. Is it possible that the holistic approach as outlined in *Seeing Without Glasses* is necessary for the overall "whole-person" shifts? Control-group subjects were later taken through exactly the same experimental program without the dedicated support, and their findings did not change significantly. These subjects were less inclined to comply with such requirements as sticking to the nutritional and exercise suggestions. Future studies can investigate this further.

The three-phase program clearly demonstrated that when persons are adequately trained and supervised, they can execute a home-based vision-fitness program. It is my desire that such home-based programs be taught to our children so that they can attain high levels of vision-fitness and perhaps permit themselves the possibility of *Seeing Without Glasses*.

Selected Bibliography

Akyol, N. *Aqueous Humor and Serum Zinc and Copper Concentrations of Patients with Glaucoma and Cataract.* British J. Ophthal. 74: 661–62, 1990.

Anderson, A. *How the Mind Heals.* Psychology Today, Dec. 1982, pp. 51–56.

Aronsfeld, G. H. *Eyesight Training and Development.* J. Am. Optom. Assoc. 7(4): 36–38, 1936.

Baldwin, W. R. *A Review of Statistical Studies of Relations Between Myopia and Ethnic, Behavioral, and Psychological Characteristics.* Am. J. Optom. Physiol. Opt. 58(7): 516–27, 1981.

Balliet, R.; Clay, A.; and Blood, K. *The Training of Visual Acuity in Myopia.* J. Am. Optom. Assoc. 53(9): 719–24, 1982.

Beach, G.; and Kavner, R. S. *Conjoint Therapy: A Cooperative Psychotherapeutic-Optometric Approach to Therapy.* J. Am. Optom. Assoc. 48(12): 1501–8, 1977.

Bell, G. *A Review of the Sclera and Its Role in Myopia.* J. Am. Optom. Assoc. 49: 1399–1403, 1978.

Bell, G. R. *The Coleman Theory of Accommodation and Its Relevance to Myopia.* J. Am. Optom. Assoc. 51(6): 582–87, 1980.

Birnbaum, M. H. *Holistic Aspects of Visual Style: A Hemispheric Model with Implications for Vision Therapy.* J. Am. Optom. Assoc. 49(10): 1133–41, 1978.

Dowis, R. T. *The Effect of a Visual Training Program on Juvenile Delinquency.* J. Am. Optom. Assoc. 48(9): 1173–76, 1193–94, 1977.

Forest, E. *Functional Vision: Its Impact on Learning.* J. Optom. Vis. Devel. 13(2): 12–15, 1982.

Francke, A. W.; and Carr, W. K. *Culture and the Development of Vision.* J. Am. Optom. Assoc. 47(1): 14–41, 1976.

Friedman, E. *Vision Training Program for Myopia Management.* Am. J. Optom. Physiol. Opt. 58(7): 546–53, 1981.

Gil, K. M.; and Collins, F. L. *Behavioral Training for Myopia: Generalization of Effects.* Behavior Res. Ther. 21(3): 269–73, 1983.

Goss, D. A. *Attempts to Reduce the Rate of Increase of Myopia in Young People: A Critical Literature Review*. Am. J. Optom. Physiol. Opt. 59(10): 828–41, 1982.

Gottlieb, R. L. *Neuropsychology of Myopia*. J. Optom. Vis. Devel. 13(1): 3–27, 1982.

Graham, C.; and Leibowitz, H. W. *The Effect of Suggestion on Visual Acuity*. Int. J. Clin. and Exp. Hypnosis 20(3): 169–86, 1972.

Greenspan, S. B. *1979 Annual Review of Literature in Developmental Optometry*. J. Optom. Vis. Devel. 10(1): 12–74, 1979.

Harris, P. A. *Myopia Control in China*. Opt. Extension Program 53, 1981.

Jensen, H. *Myopia Progression in Young School Children and Intra Ocular Pressure*. Documenta Ophthalmologica 82: 249, 1992.

Kaplan, R.-M. *Hypnosis, New Horizons for Optometry*. Rev. Optom. 115(10): 53–58, 1978.

Kaplan, R.-M. *Orthoptics or Surgery? A Case Report*. Optom. Weekly 68(39): 33–36, 1977.

Kaplan, R.-M. *Changes in Form Visual Fields in Reading Disabled Children Produced by Syntonic (Colored Light) Stimulation*. The Int. J. of Biosocial Res. 5(1): 20–33, 1983.

Kappel, G. *Cataract Prevention and Cure Research*. Opt. Extension Program 52, 1980.

Kefley, C. R. *Psychological Factors in Myopia*. J. Am. Optom. Assoc. 33(6): 833–37, 1962.

Kirshner, A. J. *Visual Training and Motivation*. J. Am. Optom. Assoc. 38(8): 641–45, 1967.

Kruger, P. B. *The Effect of Cognitive Demand on Accommodation*. Am. J. Optom. Physiol. Opt. 57(7): 440–45, 1980.

Lane, B. *Nutrition and Vision*. J. Optom. Vis. Devel. 11(3): 1–11, 1980.

Lane, B. C. *Diet and Glaucoma*. J. Am. College of Nutrition 10(5): 536, Abstract 11, Oct. 1991.

O'Toole A. J; and Kersten, D. J. *Learning to See Random Dot Stereograms*. Perceptions 21(2): 227–43, 1992.

Passo, M. S., et al. *Exercise Training Reduces Intraocular Pressure Among Subjects Suspected of Having Glaucoma*. Arch. Ophthal. 109: 1096–98, 1991.

Rutstein, R. P.; and Fuhr, P. C. *Efficacy of Stability of Amblyopia*. Therapy, Vis. Sci. 69(10): 747–54, Oct. 1992.

Whitmore, W. *Congenital and Developmental Myopia*. Eye 6: 361, 1992.

Suggested Reading

Agarwal, R. S. *Mind and Vision, Sri Aurobindo Ashram Trust*. Lotus Light (P.O. Box 2, Wilmot, WI 53192), 1978.

Aihara, Herman. *Basic Macrobiotics*. Tokyo and New York: Japan Publications, Inc., 1985.

Asher, Harry. *Experiments in Seeing*. Greenwich, Conn.: Fawcett, 1961.

Brown, Barbara. *Super Mind*. Harper Row, 1980.

Buzan, Tony. *Using Both Sides of Your Brain*. New York: E. P. Dutton, 1974.

Coca, Arthur. *The Pulse Test*. New York: Arco, 1978.

Cooper, Kenneth. *The Aerobics Way*. New York: M. Evans, 1977.

Delacato, Carl H. *The Treatment and Prevention of Reading Problems*. Springfield, Ill.: Charles C. Thomas, 1959.

Edwards, Betty. *Drawing on the Right Side of the Brain*. Los Angeles: Tarcher, 1979.

Forrest, Elliot B. *Stress and Vision*. Optometric Extension Program Foundation Inc. (2912 S. Daimler St., Santa Ana, CA 92705-5811), 1988.

Franck, Frederick. *The Zen of Seeing*. New York: Vintage Books, 1973.

Gold, Svea. *When Children Invite Child Abuse: A Search for Answers When Love Is Not Enough*. Eugene, Ore.: Fern Ridge Press, 1986.

Goldberg, Stephen. *The Four-Minute Neurological Exam*. Medmaster, 1984.

Goodrich, Janet. *Natural Vision Improvement*. Berkeley, Calif.: Celestial Arts, 1986.

Huxley, Aldous. *The Art of Seeing*. Seattle, Wash.: Montana Books, 1975.

Kaplan, Robert-Michael. *The Power Behind Your Eyes*. Inner Traditions International (One Park Street, Rochester, VT 05767), 1995.

Kavner, Richard. *Your Child's Vision and Total Vision*. Kavner Books (P.O. Box 297, Milwood, NY 10546), 1978.

Kime, Zane. *Sunlight Could Save Your Life*. Penryn, Calif.: World Health Publication, 1985.

Leviton, Richard. *Seven Steps to Better Vision*. East West/Natural Health Books (17 Station Street, Brookline, MA 02146), 1992.

Liberman, Jacob. *Light Medicine of the Future*. Santa Fe, N.M.: Bear & Co. Publishing, 1991.

Lowen, Alexander. *Bioenergetics*. New York: Penguin Books, 1975.

Mendelsohn, Robert. *Confessions of a Medical Heretic*. Chicago: Contemporary Books, 1979.

Ott, John. *Health and Light*. Old Greenwich, Conn.: Devin-Adair, 1973.

Ott, John. *Light, Radiation and You*. Old Greenwich, Conn.: Devin-Adair, 1982.

Ponder, Catherine. *Dynamic Laws of Prosperity*. Englewood Cliffs, N.J.: Prentice-Hall, 1962.

Ray, Sondra. *Loving Relationships*. Millbrae, Calif.: Celestial Arts, 1980.

Rotte, Joanna, and Koji Yamamoto. *Vision: A Holistic Guide to Healing the Eyesight*. New York: Japan Publications, 1986.

Samuels, Michael and Nancy. *Seeing with the Mind's Eye*. New York: Random House, 1975.

Schneider, Meir. *Self Healing My Life and Vision*. New York: Routledge & Kegan Paul Inc., Methuen Inc., 1987.

Scholl, Lisette. *Visionetics*. New York: Doubleday, 1978.

Shankman, Albert. *Vision Enhancement Training*. Optometric Extension Program Foundation, Inc. (2912 S. Daimler St., Santa Ana, CA 92705-5811), 1988.

Simonton, Carl O. *Getting Well Again*. New York: Bantam Books, 1980.

Smotherman, Ron. *Winning Through Enlightenment*. San Francisco: Context Publications, 1980.

Vissel, Joyce and Barry. *Models of Love: The Parent-Child Journey*. Aptos, Calif.: Ramira Publishing, 1986.

Resources

Association for Children and Adults with Learning Disabilities
4156 Library Road, Pittsburgh, PA 15234
(Parent/teacher support and network organization)

College of Optometrists in Vision Development
353 H St., Suite C, Chula Vista, CA 92010
(Referral for optometrists who provide vision-therapy services)

Optometric Extension Program Foundation, Inc.
2912 S. Daimler St., Santa Ana, CA 92705
www.healthy.net/oep
www.oep.org
(Optometrists interested in functional vision)

National Health Federation
P.O. Box 688, Monrovia, CA 91016
(Political and educational organization dedicated to protecting the health rights of the public)

American Optometric Association
243 N. Lindberg Blvd., St. Louis, MO 63141
(The most active organization for the optometric profession)

Vision-Improvement Programs and Services

As I contemplate the past fifteen years since I first published this material, I am pleased with the many letters and phone calls I have received. I realize that reading a book is one way to gain the knowledge to improve one's seeing potential. In addition, phone and e-mail consultation support programs and tools can help you make your goal a reality. My research has shown that without ongoing consultation support most people's motivation and enthusiasm decrease with time.

I will be there to help you when you make the commitment to help yourself. I have evolved a follow-up process that truly works. Once a month you phone or e-mail me for a ten- or fifteen-minute consultation. You write your questions or have them ready. Your progress and problematic areas are discussed and solutions are offered for your challenges.

After the e-mail or phone consultation you come away with renewed interest and practical pointers to continue your vision-fitness program. This process may include aspects of personal development in addition to your vision-fitness program.

In between our phone meetings you may make use of the following vision-fitness tools, depending on your diagnosed eye condition. You may also order a personalized self-healing audiotape that I can custom-design for you after a phone consultation.

I wish you well on your vision journey.

Roberto Kaplan

Near/Farsightedness
Vision-Fitness Program

Four Audiotapes: *"Seeing Without Glasses Home Training"*

These tapes take you through a sequenced adventure that helps you master the vision-fitness games while you are walking, cooking, or riding in a car. The games give you practical understanding of ways to improve your vision. The repetitious learning enables you to develop new habits of seeing clearly as you go through the developmental stages of vision improvement using one eye, partly two-eyes, and then full binocular vision. Thereafter, you play a twenty-minute maintenance audiotape to continue your progress.

Audiotape: "Relax and See"

You listen to the "Relax and See" tape during the day, before you sleep, or after a long day at work. Dr. Kaplan's calming voice guides you into a deep relaxation, while a female voice provides audible affirmation for your clear vision.

Phases One and Two Vision-Fitness Kit

This kit provides all the tools needed to train and enhance your perceptions through each eye. You use Eye-C Charts™ to monitor your flashes of clear eyesight, train yourself to let in healing color-balanced light, and patch one eye at a time and follow the swingball to synchronize your brain.

Phase Three Vision-Fitness Kit

This kit consists of materials needed for the integration phase of brain/eye re-education. A special wire is molded into the fencing game of crossing and uncrossing your eyes. The string and beads improve how your two eyes cooperate, while the integration cards permit the development of stereoscopic depth perception.

Audiotapes: "Letting Go" and either "Nearsightedness" or "Farsightedness"

Letting go of old influences that affect your ability to bring about self-healing is an integral part of your home vision-fitness program. The cells and structure of your eyes have the ability to regenerate, and it is happening all the time. Listening to the special audiotape for your specific eye condition focuses your attention on positive ways to return healthy visual function to your eyes.

Instructional Paper: "Vision Improvement after Forty" (sent electronically)

Find out about vision-enhancement techniques for restoring and increasing vision-fitness even though your eyes have changed with age. This is a special time for farsighted people to learn how to be clear and focused in their lives.

Near Eye-C Chart™

This specially designed simulated eye-training chart gives you the experience of learning to focus your mind such that your vision-fitness increases. The Near Eye-C Chart™ is laminated and contains step-by-step instructions. Many clients have reported excellent results from using this chart to measure their performance.

Pinholes

These are the glasses with small holes in them. They are one of the many tools you can use on your journey to better vision. Spend time wearing the pinholes instead of your glasses. They give added sharpness of eyesight while avoiding eyestrain. Pinholes are also available separately from Beyond Words Publishing or by e-mailing *info@beyond2020vision.com*.

Eye Disease
Vision-Fitness Program

Instructional Paper: "Food/Eating and Being Clear"

Discover how to use organic foods to create wholesome meals that sustain and bring vital vitamins and trace minerals into your eyes. This way of eating teaches you how to use food to help regenerate your eye tissue and function.

Audiotapes: "Letting Go" and special audiotapes for your eye condition (for example, "Cataracts")

Letting go of old influences that affect your ability to bring about self-healing is an integral part of your home vision program. Listening to the special audiotape for your specific eye condition focuses your attention on positive ways to return healthy visual function to your eyes.

Instructional Paper: "Light and Color for Self-Healing" (sent electronically)

Research has demonstrated that specific color frequencies programmed through the eyes have a balancing effect on the brain via the autonomic nervous system. Learn how you can use light and color to support the other elements of your self-healing program.

Color Balancing Kit™

Slip on a pair of plastic goggles housing two pairs of colored gels. These colors act as either stimulants or relaxants, depending on your needs and the colors utilized. The colored light helps your natural self-healing process and restores balance to your nervous system.

Audiotape: "Regenerate"

The cells and structure of the eyes have the ability to regenerate, and it is happening all the time. By listening to this audiotape you have the opportunity to enhance this self-healing process.

Cost of Programs and Ordering Information

Near/Farsightedness Vision-Fitness Program: $155 U.S. or $220 Cdn.
Eye Disease Vision-Fitness Program: $90 U.S. or $130 Cdn.

Prices include shipping and handling in North America; for orders to other countries please add an additional $25 U.S. or $33 Cdn. You may pay by Visa or MasterCard (charged in Canadian funds) or by check (U.S. accepted). In Canada add 7% GST; in B.C. add 7.5% PST.

Beyond 20/20 Vision®
Eckpergasse 31/7
A-1180 Wien
Austria
Phone: 011-43-676-619-2048 (from the United States and Canada)
        0043-676-619-2048 (from the United Kingdom)
Fax: 604-608-3519
E-mail: *order@beyond2020vision.com*
www.beyond2020vision.com

Personalized Self-Healing Audiotapes

A personalized self-healing audiotape can be recorded during a phone consultation with Dr. Kaplan. Provide your name, phone number, and e-mail address and request an appointment for phone consultation. Dr. Kaplan will spend fifteen minutes asking you questions in preparation to custom-design your healing tape that will focus on the issues in your eyes and life that will benefit from healing.

Seeing Without Glasses
The Eye Seminar

The Eye Seminar™ is an annual seven-day retreat event held in Europe, Canada, or the United States. It uses the *Seeing Without Glasses* books, tapes, and kits developed by Dr. Kaplan as tools for a deep healing of your eyes and your life. The retreat is ideal for people who wish to immerse themselves in a deeper experience of enhancing their vision. In addition, if you are interested in assisting others in improving their vision-fitness, you can also use the retreat as an opportunity to gain competencies to become a certified vision educator. Vision education is a growing discipline and profession throughout the world, and the demand for certified persons is increasing. The certification can also be accomplished with the **Healthy Eyes Home-Study Course** developed by Dr. Kaplan.

Dr. Kaplan also teaches **The Love Seminar™**, an in-depth seven-day retreat, with his wife, Gabriela Kaplan.

Contact Information

Dr. Roberto Kaplan
Eckpergasse 31/7
A-1180 Wien
Austria
Phone: 011-43-676-619-2048 (from the United States and Canada)
   0043-676-619-2048 (from the United Kingdom)
Fax: 604-608-3519
E-mail: *robertocap@utanet.at*
www.robertokaplan.com

Referral Directory

If you would like to contact a trained vision educator you can contact the following people:

Master Practitioners of Integrated Vision Therapy (Most Advanced Certification)

AUSTRIA
Gabriela Kaplan
Eckpergasse 31/7
1180-Wien
Phone/fax: 0043-1-478-8437
E-mail: *gabriela.kaplan@happyandhealthy.at*
www.happyandhealthy.at

Dr. Roberto Kaplan
Eckpergasse 31/7
1180-Wien
Phone: 011-43-676-619-2048 (from the United States and Canada)
         0043-676-619-2048 (from the United Kingdom)
Fax: 604-608-3519
E-mail: *robertokap@utanet.at*
www.robertokaplan.com

Practitioners of Integrated Vision Therapy (Advanced Certification)

AUSTRALIA
John Palassis
Ezekiel Optometrists
43 Outram St.
West Perth, 6005
Western Australia

Phone: 61 8 9322 4443
Fax: 61 8 9322 3826
E-mail: *john@ezeoptom.com* or *palassis@iinet.net.au*

Certified Vision Educators

AUSTRIA
Hilde Enzinger
Emzersberg 182
A-5303 Thalgau
Phone: 06235-6266
E-mail: *hilde.enzinger@utanet.at*

Maria Iwan
Nationalparksiedlung 59/1/6
A-7132 Frauenkirchen
Phone: 02172-2627

Eva Thilde Liwanetz
Kriehubergasse 29/6
A 1050 Wien
Phone 0043 (0)664 33 89 171
E-mail: *eva.thilde@gmx.at*
www.gesundheit.web.com

Barbara Moshammer
Neudorfegg 40 A
A-8522 Groß St. Florian
Phone: 03464-8794
E-mail: *conservation.eng@sime.com*

Evi Sitton
Reinhold Diessnerstr. 8
2100 Korneuberg
Phone: 0043 2262-62145
Fax: 0043 699-106 30 278
E-mail: *evi.sitton@i-one.at*

Lifebalance Zentrum
Erbpostgasse 7
1210 Wien
Phone: 43-1-292 88 88
E-mail: *lifebalance@aon.at*
www.lifebalance.at

CANADA
Damara Sylvester
1466 Gladstone Ave.
Victoria, B.C. V8R 1S3
Phone: 250-595-1051
E-mail: *damsylfly@excite.com*

Isabella Pe Le Hentsch
E-mail: *pelelight@comperserve.com*

Anne Marie Konas
Vancouver, B.C.
Phone: 604-871-3035
E-mail: *amkonas@hotmail.com*

FRANCE
Agnes Glaise
24 Rue Massena
0600 Nice
Phone: 0033 06 686 006847
E-mail: *aglaise@yahoo.com*

GERMANY
Ursula Buechler
Theodolindenplatz 5
81545 Munchen
Phone: 089-648531
E-mail: *opticartbuechler@t-online.de*

Christine Graef
Brönnerstraße 26
D-60313 Frankfurt/Main
Phone: 0049-(0)172-6588711
E-mail: *christine.graef@accenture.com*

Uta Halm
Rehmstr. 51
49080 Osnabruck
Phone: 0541/21670
E-mail: *utahalm@hotmail.com*

Karl-Heinz Hengstler
Hinterbergstraße 17
D-65207 Wiesbaden
Phone: 0611-9507041
Fax: 0611-9507042
E-mail: *hengstler.gap@gmx.de*

Ulrike Jung
Nahest 9
Mainz 55118
E-mail: *ulrike.jung@t-online.de*

Christine Klein
Steubenstraße 73 A
D-63743 Aschaffenburg
Phone: 0049-6021-91652
Fax: 0049-172-6005863
Mobile: 0049-6021-91652

Dr. Andrea Lusser
Steinackerstraße 8
D-79117 Freiburg
Phone: 0049-(0)761-65513
Fax: 0049-(0)761-65514
E-mail: *andrea.lusser@web.de*

Angelika Maybusch
Obernheideweg 46
D-33106 Paderborn
Phone: 05254-67372

Petra Renkel
Zweigstr. 24
42657 Solingen
Phone: 0212/817986

Baerbel Schroeder
Gros ringmar 11
D-27211 Bassum
Phone: 04241-970053
E-mail: *hygieia@gmx.de*

Ingrid Schuchardt
Richard Wagnerstraße 38
D-45128 Essen
Phone: 0201-2200855

Fax: 0201-2438909
E-mail: *ingrid.schuchardt@t-online.de*

Peter Andreas Thaler
E-mail: *thalerandreas@hotmail.com*

Elke Willutzki
Rahmer Str. 273
44369 Dortmund
Phone: 0231/673999
Fax: 0231/674944
E-mail: *elke.w@t-online.de*

Marianne Witt
Heerdestr. 20
D-48149 Muenster
Phone: 0251/274417

GREAT BRITAIN
Angela Eckles
62 Highfield Road
Dartford, Kent
DA1 2JJ
Phone: 0044 01322 270044
E-mail: *angela@angelco.fsnet.co.uk*

IRELAND
Brian Smith
60 Heather View Drive
Aylesbury
Dublin 24
Phone: +353 1 4521 255

NEW ZEALAND
Adriana Young (optometrist)
P.O. Box 74569
Market Road
Auckland, 1135
Phone/fax: 64 9 529 5432
E-mail: *y_adrian@hotmail.com*

SPAIN
Amelia Salvador (ophthalmologist)
Peña del Aguila 12
Denia 03700 (Alicante)
E-mail: *asalvadorvi@coma.es*

SWITZERLAND
Joseph Fasel (optometrist)
Rue St. Pierre 10
Case postale 302
CH-1701 Fribourg-Schweiz
Phone: 0041-26322-7876
E-mail: *jfaseloptometrie@bluewin.ch*

UNITED STATES
Sandra Merideth, M.F.A.
A Life with a View
6 Lucero Road
Santa Fe, NM 87505
Phone: 505-466-6413
E-mail: *lifeview360@hotmail.com*

C. J. Wilson
275 S. French Broad Ave.
Asheville, NC 28753
Phone: 828-281-3230
E-mail: *cjwilson@madison.main.nc.us*

Jillane Hinds
E-mail: *roadangel1@hotmail.com*

Index

Note: Vision games appear in boldface

Fovea: exercises for, 27, 30, 110–11, 113–19; foveal (focused looking) state, 27, 31–34, 35–36, 67; function of, 27; nutrition for, 43; sunlight and, 95. *See also* Retina; Visual style

Glaucoma: mind's-eye perception and, 52; pinholes for, 153–54; rehabilitation for, 165; sunlight as treatment for, 25

Goal-setting, 85–88, 100–102

Healing. *See* Mind's-eye perception

Imaging game, 144–45

Iris: exercises for, 30, 122–24; function of, 25. *See also* Light

Lazy eye, 52, 70

Left-eye perception. *See* Coordination, two-eyed

Lens and ciliary muscle: exercises for, 26–27, 30, 77–78; function of, 26; nutrition for, 39, 41–42, 43; overstraining of, 29, 32. *See also* Visual style

Lens prescriptions: for astigmatism, 4–5, 14; for farsightedness, 14; full-strength, 5, 14, 15–16; near-distance (focusing or stress-relieving), 16; for nearsightedness, 5, 14; single-eye test for, 5. *See also* Corrective lenses; Vision-fitness: lenses

Light. *See also* Glaucoma
—artificial: sources for, 25–26, 122; use with vision games, 106, 122–24
—full-spectrum (sunlight): value of, 25–26, 95, 166
—**Lighting game**, 25–26, 122–24

Macula, 43. *See also* Fovea

Macular degeneration, 52; pinholes for, 153–54; rehabilitation for, 165

Maintenance program, 145

Marching game, 129–30

Massage. *See* Shoulder and neck massage game

Mind's-eye perception. *See also* Coordination, two-eyed; Eye/brain connection; Visual style
—astigmatism and, 51, 59
—case histories, 49, 50–51, 57–59
—as cause of eye problems, 48–52, 55–60, 61–65, 162–63, 167
—chart: *Perceptual Understanding of Various Eye Conditions*, 51–52
—emotions of anger and fear, 56–57, 61–65
—exercises: **Arrows game**, 78–80; **Mind's eye game**, 78; **Nose pencil game**, 120–21; **Painting/yawning game**, 111–13; **Trampoline game**, 61–63, 78, 130; **Visual mapping game**, 64
—and peripheral vision, 49
—and sexual/visual orientation, 68–69
—and vision-fitness lenses, 65

Muscles, outside eye: exercises for, 28–29, 127–29; function of, 23

Nearsightedness: definition of, 4; mind's-eye perception and, 51, 57–59, 65; physical causes of, 10–11, 78; pinholes for, 148, 152; statistics on, xiii, 9, 11; vision games for, 100

Beyond Words Publishing, Inc.

OUR CORPORATE MISSION

Inspire to Integrity

OUR DECLARED VALUES

We give to all of life as life has given us.

We honor all relationships.

Trust and stewardship are integral to fulfilling dreams.

Collaboration is essential to create miracles.

Creativity and aesthetics nourish the soul.

Unlimited thinking is fundamental.

Living your passion is vital.

Joy and humor open our hearts to growth.

It is important to remind ourselves of love.

To order or to request a catalog, contact
Beyond Words Publishing, Inc.
20827 N.W. Cornell Road, Suite 500
Hillsboro, OR 97124-9808
503-531-8700

You can also visit our Web site at *www.beyondword.com*
or e-mail us at *info@beyondword.com*.